Storytelling with Data in Healthcare

With the constant evolution of change in healthcare from both a technology and governmental perspective, it is imperative to take a step back and view the big picture. Relying on hunches or beliefs is no longer sustainable, so avoid jumping to conclusions and making decisions without thoroughly understanding the statistics being analyzed. The triple aim of statistics is a conceptual model laying the foundation for improving healthcare outcomes through statistics. This foundation is: know your numbers; develop behavioral interventions; and set goals to drive change.

With the availability of electronic data sources, the quantity and quality of data have grown exponentially to the point of information overload. Translating all this data into words that tell a meaningful story is overwhelming. This book takes the reader on a journey that navigates through this data to tell a story that everyone can understand and use to drive improvement. Readers will learn to tell a narrative story based on data, to develop creative, innovative, and effective solutions to improve processes and outcomes utilizing the authors' tools. Topics include mortality and readmission, patient experience, patient safety survey, governmental initiatives, CMS Star Rating, and Hospital Compare.

Storytelling with Data in Healthcare combines methodology and statistics in the same course material, making it coherent and easier to put into practice. It uses storytelling as a tool for knowledge acquisition and retention and will be valuable for courses in nursing schools, medical schools, pharmacy schools, or any healthcare profession that has a research design or statistics course offered to students. The book will be of interest to researchers, academics, healthcare professionals, and students in the fields of healthcare management and operations as well as statistics and data visualization.

Kevin D. Masick is the Owner/Principal Consultant at Masick Consulting, LLC.

Eric Bouillon is a Consultant at Masick Consulting, LLC.

Storytelling with Data in Healthcare

Kevin D. Masick and Eric Bouillon

Routledge
Taylor & Francis Group

NEW YORK AND LONDON

First published 2021
by Routledge
52 Vanderbilt Avenue, New York, NY 10017

and by Routledge
2 Park Square, Milton Park, Abingdon, Oxon OX14 4RN

Routledge is an imprint of the Taylor & Francis Group, an informa business

© 2021 Taylor & Francis

Library of Congress Cataloging-in-Publication Data
A catalog record for this title has been requested

ISBN: 978-0-367-46144-7 (hbk)
ISBN: 978-0-367-89877-9 (pbk)
ISBN: 978-1-003-02721-8 (ebk)

Typeset in Bembo Std
by Newgen Publishing UK

Contents

Author biography

Kevin Masick

Kevin is a leader, author, speaker, consultant, research methodologist, and statistical expert with over 15 years of experience in healthcare and academia. As a healthcare leader, he has worked for three healthcare systems in human resources, quality management, and strategic planning where he has led a team of healthcare professionals in improving healthcare outcomes through innovative dashboards, analytics, research, and education. In academia, he has taught at five universities in both the business school and psychology department, teaching in-person and online undergraduate and graduate courses in research methodology and statistics. He has chaired, mentored, and served as an outside reader for more than 60 doctoral dissertations, published in peer-reviewed journals, spoke and presented at professional conferences, sat on career panels, and published an advanced research methods textbook. In addition to his full-time work, he is the owner of and principal consultant at Masick Consulting, LLC. He received his Ph.D. in applied organizational psychology and master's in industrial/organizational psychology both from Hofstra University and his bachelor's degree in psychology from SUNY Albany.

Eric Bouillon

Eric has 4 years of consulting experience at Masick Consulting, LLC. He uses his expertise in research design and statistics to coach doctoral students. He has also worked with Kevin to develop an online and in-person training program to help healthcare employees learn how to interpret and utilize statistics in practice. Recently, while writing this book, Eric was finishing up his Ph.D. at Hofstra University in organizational psychology. His dissertation focused on creating a scale that utilized psychometric and scale development best practices to measure how well individuals use statistics to find data-driven solutions in organizations. Most recently, Eric has branched out of academia and was hired as a people scientist at a recruitments firm to help develop tailored assessments for selection. He also spearheaded the development of a new tool that measures organizational purpose through psychometric testing. He received his Ph.D. in applied organizational psychology and master's in industrial/organizational psychology both from Hofstra University and bachelor's degree in psychology from Northeastern University.

Preface

Here are some notes from Kevin regarding the idea behind this book. As I sit here and begin to write this book, I think back on how I arrived at the place I'm supposed to be and wonder if I'll ever get to where I want to be. Throughout the journey of writing this book, I have kept notes highlighting my journey. Inspiration comes from experiences and a lot of my experiences have altered the way I approach my professional and personal life. Consider these lessons learned.

One particular experience that I reflect on is sitting on career panels. A common question that I've been asked on these panels is how I ended up where I am in my career. The answer is that I don't really know. Throughout my college education, I was convinced that, based on my limited work experience, healthcare or research were two areas where I didn't want to work. The irony is that I am in healthcare and I conduct research. Lesson learned: as clichéd as it may sound, sometimes you don't choose your career; your career chooses you. My career has spanned both academia and professional practice simultaneously. I strongly believe that both careers have shaped who I have become. Lesson learned: being in academia, I reflect on the concept that I never want to forget what it's like to be a student learning something for the first time. As a professional, I can bring valuable real-life examples in practice to the classroom and academic rigor into a professional environment.

Throughout my time in healthcare, I've learned that not everyone looks at numbers and statistics the same way that I do. When I look at graphs or statistics I see a story where numbers translate into words like pictures. Lesson learned: you're probably familiar with the expression that a picture is worth a thousand words. I'll modify that statement with "numbers are worth a thousand words." If I can teach someone a skill that saves them time and allows them to connect the dots, then I consider it a success. My lifelong goal is to teach others how to look at numbers in a different way and to give a new meaning to the word statistics. What if statistics is just like learning a second language? Within this book, I wanted to infuse industrial/organizational psychology, statistics, research methodology, and healthcare into a toolkit to help you translate numbers into actionable results. I thank you for deciding to take this journey with me and give me a second chance to make a first impression with statistics.

Now that this book is finished, I can truly say that I am extremely proud of what it has turned into. This journey started as an idea in early 2015. I wrote the initial draft of the entire book in 2 months, but took a hiatus in 2018 during my transition from New York to Florida. It has been sitting on the back burner while I re-aligned my personal and professional life. It's something that I always thought about and I'm ecstatic to put it out there. There's definitely been bumps in the road and many opportunities to abandon the idea. It's much easier to give up than to continue on. Lesson learned: when you believe in something, stick with it. Perseverance and dedication can push you to the finish line.

I really hope you enjoy and learn from this book. It has truly taught me many lessons along the way, but perhaps the most important lesson was that the journey is more important than the destination.

Acknowledgments

Kevin Masick

Writing a book is no easy task. There are a lot of individuals involved in the process who have guided me, shaped me, kept me sane, and encouraged me along the way. First and foremost, I would like to thank Rob Tursi-Masick for always being there for me and providing feedback in the beginning stages of this journey. Being able to bounce initial ideas off you was extremely helpful in shaping the final product. I'll do my best to keep my rambling to a minimum! I want to thank my daughter, Madeline Tursi-Masick, for pulling me away from the book to spend some much-needed quality family time to then drive me nuts and make me want to continue writing. I would also like to acknowledge and thank my mom, Nancy Masick, for all her support over the years.

Professionally, I owe a lot of thanks to those individuals I have spoken to over the years for their help and guidance and for being there to pass along ideas as I started this journey. I remember the day like it was yesterday. On March 16, 2018, I had the opportunity to sit down with Carolyn Sweetapple for breakfast. I'll never forget driving to the diner telling myself not to get emotional about how you helped change my life, but it didn't work. You are a true inspiration and I thank you immensely for your support and guidance. It means more to me than you will ever know. As I said then, you are the inspiration behind writing this book. I am honored to call you a friend.

I owe a lot of gratitude to Kathy Gallo for truly listening and encouraging me to further develop my idea and write this book. You were able to see my vision when it wasn't 100% clear to me.

Marty Doefler – every once in a while you cross paths with someone who has a tremendous impact on your life. I'm not sure if I ever told you how much your support and actions have helped me gain confidence in my work. You have an amazing gift of connecting with anyone you encounter. It means a lot to have the support and encouragement from someone like you. You really are truly a one-of-a-kind inspirational leader. You have said in the past to "never let great get in the way of good." It's an important reminder that while we may strive for perfection, it must not get in the way of accomplishing your goal.

I was blessed to be surrounded by an amazing group of nurses that I have learned so much from. With your help and knowledge, I feel like I have a greater understanding of healthcare quality. I cannot thank you enough, Anne Marie

Fried, Isabel Friedman, Pat Hogan, and Sue Dries. Anne Marie, you have always believed in me and helped me succeed along the way. I appreciate your willingness to connect me to the right people to make my dream come true. As an aside, Greg and I think it's your time to go on this journey and write your book! Issie, I really appreciate you seeing more in me than I often see in myself. Thank you for always being a friend and lending an ear. Pat, there are no words to describe you. I always felt at ease talking to you about anything and everything. Thank you for your guidance and wisdom. Sue, I'm very appreciative of all those philosophical conversations we had. You definitely opened my eyes and forced me to think in different ways.

Yosef Dlugacz, thank you for teaching me about healthcare quality, resident education, and the importance of using data to drive decisions. Marcella De Geronimo, thank you for being the best boss and mentor I have ever had. It wasn't an easy decision to move from New York to Florida, but you always supported, encouraged, and believed in me. Rose Linton, Larry Lutsky, and Stan Cho: we had a lot of great times working together. I appreciate the candid conversations and early feedback you had provided me. Furthermore, Larry Lutsky, you are truly a blessing. Your wisdom and knowledge of just about anything are amazing. Keep writing those short stories; I really enjoy reading them! Alice Greenwood, your candor and innate ability to transform my writing over the years into a beautiful masterpiece have been a blessing. I appreciate your early feedback and comments on the book. I still find myself thinking and saying out loud, "What would Alice say?"

I would also like to acknowledge and thank the Healthcare Association of New York State (HANYS), specifically Mason Fornado, for their willingness to allow me to incorporate their Centers for Medicare/Medicaid Services (CMS) Star Rating dashboard into my book. I want to thank Christine Seery and Jenny Amarando for reading through earlier drafts of this book and providing valuable feedback along the way. I also owe a lot of gratitude to Mike Burroughs. He has been instrumental in bringing my visual ideas to life, beginning with the cover design and all graphics in the book. No matter how crazy or obscure my ideas were he was able to visualize them in ways I never thought possible. His work is outstanding and he truly collaborates with you to create amazing visuals. Visit his website for other examples: www.mikeburroughsdesign.com/. Last but not least, I'd like to acknowledge and thank my co-author Eric Bouillon. Thank you for those random conversations about how to enhance this book. It's been a pleasure writing this with you and I look forward to the next journey.

Eric Bouillon

I would just very quickly like to thank my parents who have always supported me throughout the years. Without them none of what I am doing would be possible so thank you for all that you have given me. Kevin Masick, my advisor and co-author: thank you for all the help you have given me these past few years. Your guidance and mentorship have helped tremendously and I am grateful for your friendship.

1 Introduction

"Bridging your analytical left brain with your artistic right brain"

Introduction

Now that you know more about us, let's start our journey together to build or enhance your skill set to be more comfortable and confident with interpreting/presenting statistics and leveraging statistics to drive change. Think about your response to the question: "Does the idea of analyzing statistics or presenting statistics make you nervous?" If you are hesitant on standing in front of your peers to explain data or drive home a message using statistics, then you're not alone. You're not alone with feelings of anxiety or fear while presenting statistics. Statistics is a language itself and one that is not always easily understood or spoken. Sure, it's possible to push through the presentation, but you risk someone not understanding or asking a question you don't know the answer to. Our goal throughout this journey is to teach skills to enhance your confidence when presenting statistics. We want to treat this opportunity as a second chance to make a first impression with statistics. We want to teach you the language of statistics that will transform numbers to life through storytelling.

The beginning of every story starts with knowing your numbers. You may think you know your numbers and data, but simply looking at a number doesn't indicate knowledge of the analysis or method used to derive those results. Think of the most recent presentation that you either presented or listened to that involved data. Did the presentation go well? Was the message clear and effective? Was everything known about the calculation of the numerator, denominator, and the rate/index/ratio? Did you know/understand the methodology used to arrive at those numbers? Do you know what to do to implement change? Did the presentation give the audience that "aha" moment when the light bulb went on and they knew what to do next? If you said "no" to at least one of those questions, then you're in the right place.

The goal by the end of this book is to enhance or fine tune your skills by incorporating techniques/tools to effectively explain statistics and leverage the power of storytelling with data. In reflecting back to sitting in a high school math class, we wondered how it was possible to multiply or add letters in an equation. The concept of multiplying various letters or having a letter mean something other than the ones used to create words that make up sentences is confusing. When looking at art or a photograph and feelingan emotional connection, why is it possible to describe how you feel in words? If a picture is worth a thousand words, then why can't numbers be? Thinking about the relationship between numbers and how they translate to words is complex. Part of the complexity may be a result of the left side of the brain being analytical and logical and the right side of the brain being creative and innovative. Storytelling with statistics is when the left side of the brain invades the right side.

In reflecting on a personal experience during a presentation in a high school math class, students were presented the challenge of using pictures to tell a story. Students were shown a picture of Cinderella's castle in Walt Disney World, an image of the Rorschach ink blot test, and then a control chart. A lively discussion of Walt Disney World ensued with many different personal and emotional stories. The Rorschach inkblot generated conversations and laughs where students were still able to see the story within an abstract image. Then it happened. The deafening silence that creates a sense of feeling uncomfortable. The presence of a control chart caused the room to go immediately silent with no student making eye contact for fear of being randomly called on to answer a question when they didn't know the answer. In our minds, we wondered why and how it was possible to go from genuine enthusiasm to laughter to pure fear and anxiety with three different pictures. All three images capture a moment in time when the only change is the content of the image. Why can't all images or pictures capture the same enthusiasm as Cinderella's castle or a Rorschach test? Is it a fear of the unknown or lack of confidence in how to analyze an image? We subsequently presented the same story to healthcare professionals, healthcare technology leaders, and a group of organizational professionals, with similar results.

At this moment, we realized that not everyone sees statistics as both an art and a science – the analytical science behind the statistical calculations and the art to transform statistics into a language that brings the data to life. Statistics as a science is the analytical aspect of using numbers to solve problems or answer questions. Statistics as an art is transforming these numbers into words to create an effective story used to drive change. This is exactly what we *hope to* will do! Throughout the rest of our journey together we are going to teach you skills to speak the language of statistics. Before we begin, let's reflect on setting the stage of where we are at this present moment.

Evolution of Healthcare Analytics

Years ago decisions either relied on presenting averages or percentages to demonstrate outcomes or were made using hunches, beliefs, or previous experience. At this time statistics were used to monitor compliance **metrics** over time. While it is important to monitor compliance, changes in reimbursement and accountability force organizations to utilize performance-based metrics. Part of this drive is attributed to continual change in technology that has given us access to data within healthcare that wasn't attainable in the past. Other drives are to reduce cost and improve accountability for providing care along the entire continuum.

Focusing on the facts presented is the current and future best practice of making decisions to drive sustainable change. Healthcare data has evolved, and leaders are more sophisticated by asking more challenging questions, which require advanced statistics beyond percentages or means. Questions being asked require *p* values to compare groups or use advanced statistical models to predict outcomes or combine metrics for an overall comparative rating or leverage the power of technology for machine learning/artificial intelligence. Statistics are necessary to understand the significance of interventions and how to improve care. This evolution towards big data, predictive modeling, artificial intelligence, natural language processing, or machine learning in healthcare is inevitable and already happening.

Healthcare is a complex environment and advances in technology, governmental regulatory agencies, and human interaction, where individuals often have a split second to make decisions, create a multitude of potential red flags for effectively changing behavior. Care is not only provided in a hospital. Patients are treated in multiple settings, such as: ambulatory surgery, clinics, urgent care, physician offices, ambulances, nursing homes, home, free-standing emergency departments, or any public location. Regardless of where care is delivered, metrics exist to measure performance. Change occurs quickly and frequently in healthcare, as new technologies and patient care techniques are being researched and implemented all the time. As a healthcare professional, you not only have to know the clinical side to patient care, but also need to be aware of issues that may be beyond your control.

The federal government, along with the Centers for Medicare/Medicaid Services (CMS) and the Joint Commission, is becoming stricter in the delivery of healthcare by implementing financial penalties based on performance. Likewise, there may be state regulatory agencies, like the State Department of Health, healthcare lobbying organizations, and many outside agencies that provide data to the public (i.e., Press Ganey, Centers for Disease Control, Agency for Healthcare Research and Quality (AHRQ), etc.). There are many healthcare initiatives that must be taken into consideration and monitored, like Pay 4 Performance, Partnership for Patients, Value-Based Purchasing (VBP), Bundled Payments, CMS Star Rating, Affordable Care Act (ACA), Leapfrog, US News, and World Reports. All of these initiatives can be overwhelming to know and understand, since minimal focus during your education may be on statistics or research methodology.

As a healthcare professional, do you feel overwhelmed by the volume of metrics that you are required to monitor? Are you faced with doing more with less? Do you feel that you are being told to improve patient care and the overall patient experience while driving down cost and remaining efficient? Does the Triple Aim sound familiar? The Triple Aim was initiated by the Institute for Healthcare Improvement (IHI) to simultaneously improve the patient experience, improve the health of populations, and reduce cost (www.ihi.org). How easy is it for you to know the details on all metrics of the CMS Star system, the hundreds of metrics requiring improvement in your organization, or the financial penalty you will be hit with? This seemingly impossible task can be possible with the right tools and techniques.

For every intervention developed, every goal achieved, every patient experience improved, every financial incentive earned, know that everyone else will continue to improve, so goals set today may not be sufficient tomorrow. We are all on the same trajectory towards improving the overall patient experience, improving care, and decreasing cost. The competition and stakes get higher with every national benchmark you achieve and every goal you exceed. As the world continues to improve, the chance of becoming the top performer seems out of reach. So you've decreased mortality rates by 50%? Well, that 50% reduction over the course of 5 years may have been fantastic, but to get to the top you have to cut it by 50% again. The never-ending battle to become #1 becomes increasingly difficult when the target moves.

Despite the constant determination to get to the top, the basic principles at the bottom don't change. Analyzing data methodologically ensures a greater understanding and appreciation of what you're looking at and provides the depth of knowledge to internalize results and ask the right questions. Remember, the pathway to storytelling with data begins with STATISTICS. Never lose sight of the purpose of what you are trying to do. Every statistical analysis begins with a foundation that we call the Three Pillars of Statistics (Figure 1.1).

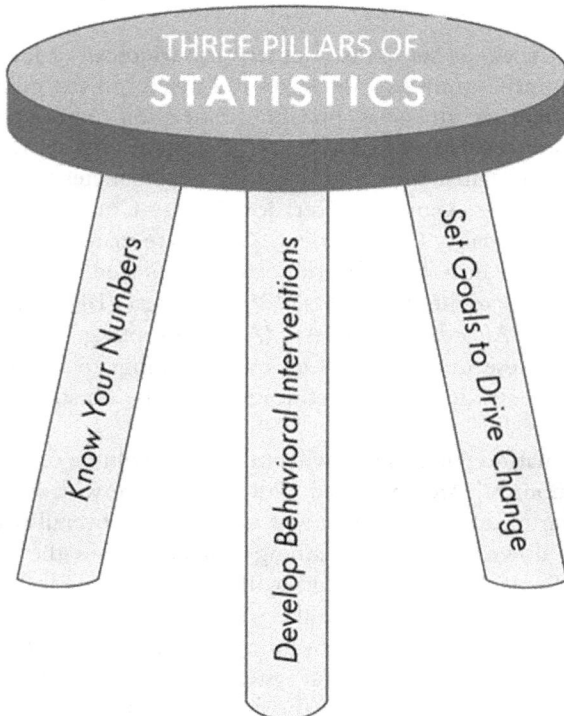

Figure 1.1 Three Pillars of Statistics.

1. Know your numbers – critically think, evaluate, and DEFINE statistics.
2. Develop behavioral interventions – know how you're being measured and create processes to change behavior through a focus on the FACTS.
3. Set goals to drive change – STOP to develop achievable methodological goals to drive change.

Change starts with a solid foundation. Removing any one leg from the stool results in the stool falling over. The Three Pillars of Statistics is our conceptual framework that utilizes out toolkit to drive and develop critical thinking, systematic thinking, and statistical agility. We created tools to aid in critical thinking. We used research methodology to guide the development of our STATISTICS model to encourage systematic thinking. We intertwined statistics with applied healthcare examples to enhance statistical agility for storytelling.

Know Your Numbers

One critical aspect of any statistical analysis is to know your numbers. Some people may think that knowing numbers means knowing a mortality rate, infection rate, readmission rate, or most recent patient satisfaction score. There is more to a number than the value itself. For example, a 12.7% mortality rate calculated by your organization is likely a raw rate while a 12.7% mortality rate provided by CMS is a risk-adjusted rate. Both rates may be the same, but their interpretation is different. Every number is comprised of a formula used to calculate a raw rate (i.e., an actual observed rate), a risk-adjusted index/ratio (i.e., a logistic regression modeling technique), or any other calculation that you can think of (i.e., confidence interval, odds ratio, percentile ranks, standard deviation, etc.). Every value has a theory or rationale behind the calculation. Taking a step back to understand this methodology provides a greater appreciation and internalization of the data.

Within every metric, there is a methodology used to derive that number. Breaking apart formulas and understanding the methodology provide a clearer picture of what is measured. A common statistical term, **standard deviation** is a measure of variability around the mean or how much variation there is within a metric (see Figure 1.2 for the formula). Pay careful attention to the letter n in the formula as that is the sample size. This is important for two reasons: (1) a larger sample size equals a lower standard deviation; and (2) a smaller sample size equals a

$$s = \sqrt{\frac{\sum(x - \bar{x})^2}{n - 1}}$$

Figure 1.2 Standard Deviation.

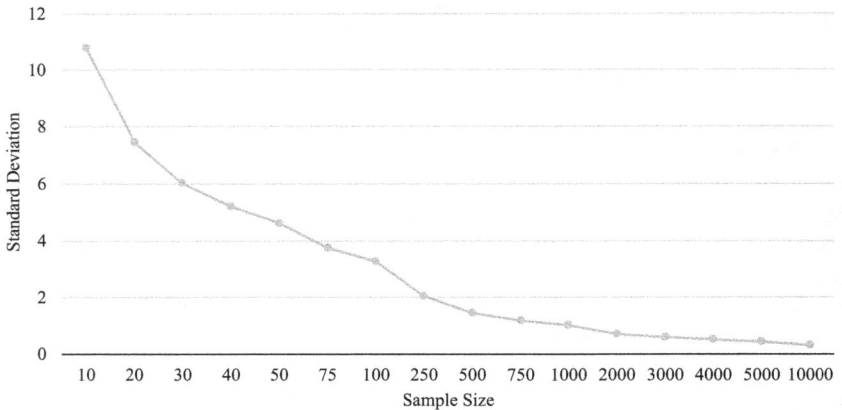

Figure 1.3 Standard Deviation by Sample Size.

larger standard deviation. Figure 1.3 is a graphical representation depicting changes in standard deviation based on sample size. This is an important factor when analyzing any data involving standard deviation (i.e., a control chart), because additional insights or stories can emerge.

Develop Behavioral Interventions

In addition to knowing your numbers, an effective way to hit moving targets is to develop behavioral interventions to drive sustainable change. Changing behavior is hard, but understanding past behavior is the best predictor of future performance (Wernimont & Campbell, 1968). Understanding how to change behavior begins with understanding change. This spectrum of change ranges from laggards (those resistant in their response to change) to early adopters (those quick to respond to change) (Rogers, 2010). There is an equally small percentage of people who both love and hate change, with more than 75% falling somewhere in the middle. One way to implement change is to seek out early adopters and eventually, if the change works, others come around and adopt it. If it doesn't, then think about why some behavioral interventions work and others don't. Was it the wrong focus on the right problem? Was it the right focus on the wrong problem? Were there not enough early adopters? Did the intervention stop when the individual implementing the change left the organization? Was the intervention not tied to a process that impacts behavioral change? Was the intervention aimed at impacting performance metrics that were part of the change? Did someone create a heuristic to complete a process faster? From a psychological perspective, we are creatures of habit. We may do things for the sake of doing it without understanding why. Then someone comes in and creates disruptive change, so we decide to resist without having an open mind.

At some point, we have been at that place where we said: "I implemented a program to address _____ (any metric), but my metric isn't improving." Taking a step back to understand the methodology of the purpose of intervention and what metrics were measured to improve is the first step to understanding why the program did not work. For example, maybe a program was implemented to improve the overall likelihood to recommend patient experience measures. Now, what behavioral intervention was implemented to impact this change? The answer to this question doesn't matter. What matters is what you believe patients are thinking about when they are asked to recommend. That statement is often followed by blank stares with an occasional: "I really don't know what the patient is recommending, but I think this is what they want." *Thinking* and *knowing* are two completely different constructs. So the new question would be, "How does the *patient* define likelihood to recommend?" (By which we mean patients' perception of whether or not they are going to say good things about an organization and encourage others to go there.) How can a program improve likelihood to recommend when you haven't asked the patient what they are recommending? Suddenly, a sense of excitement about the implemented program disappears. This methodological thinking can help to approach every analytical situation in the same way. The moral of the story is: when improving a metric, an intervention must be designed around how that metric is being measured. Incorporating theory with practice, research methodology with understanding definitions, and statistics with storytelling can help with changing culture, improving behavior, and driving change through building or enhancing your skill set, so you can be more confident with internalizing statistics.

Set Goals to Drive Change

The last concept of the Three Pillars of Statistics is driving change – one of the more challenging pillars. Having goals to achieve can drive accountability for improvement. Goal-setting theory and self-regulation, both popular theories in the industrial/organizational psychology literature, are aimed at understanding how to maximize goal setting (Bandura, 1991; Locke & Latham, 1990). Keep in mind these concepts are theories, which means they do not discuss any fundamental laws on how to set goals. The goal you set is up to you, but there is literature to support that setting appropriate goals can maximize change initiatives.

Consider the following scenario where the purpose was to set annual goals for 3 years, which are referred to as Year A, Year B, and Year C. Year A is treated as the baseline as it's already known. For argument's sake, the annual rate was 4.3% (the actual metric is irrelevant for this illustration). A lower rate for this metric is desirable, so for Year B a goal of 4.0% was set. At the end of Year B, the goal wasn't met as performance was worse than expected and the actual rate was 5.1%. Given this information, the question is: what should the goal for Year C be? Year B goal (4.0%) was calculated based on using baseline data from Year A. If Year C goal is set the same way Year B was, then it would be calculated based on Year B performance. Using baseline data from a poorly performing year (Year B) would result in a higher Year C goal. This approach would reward poor performance.

If the initial 4.0% goal set for Year B was used again for Year C, despite worse performance in Year B, then this may not be a feasible goal to achieve for Year C. This approach sets an unattainable goal, so there may be an unwillingness to work towards that goal.

So how should goals be set? Should the focus be on goal-setting theory? Should the focus be on practical solutions with no methodology or statistical rigor? Should the focus be on calculating a percent reduction or statistical model? Some goals are set by calculating a percent reduction (i.e., 2.5%) on baseline data or attempting to utilize statistical techniques (i.e., regression) to enhance the methodological rigor to set goals. Taking a step back and examining the desired direction of change and focusing on the methodology may shed light on the situation. Is a 2.5% reduction in baseline data a reasonable goal? Mathematically, a 2.5% reduction on a 1.7% baseline data would mean the new goal is 1.65%, which would round to 1.7%.

Utilizing statistical techniques to set a goal may not be ideal, because there are many variables that impact the metric. Relying on theory or statistics alone may not be enough to set goals. Analyzing the methodology and statistical concepts behind the calculation of your numbers can shed light on setting an appropriate goal. Setting goals is hard and it's important to take a step back to think about the most appropriate approach. A reasonable goal may utilize statistical techniques or reduce baseline data by a certain percentage or a combination of both.

A goal should be set to make us aware of where we need to be in order to challenge us to improve. Imagine if you never had goals in life. What would you be doing? To begin to approach this complex issue, step back and think about what you want to accomplish. First, define what the goal is. Is the goal to reduce mortality? Improve satisfaction scores? Stay out of financial penalties? Improve employee engagement? Empower others? Every goal you set must be carefully thought out.

As a healthcare professional, there are benefits to incorporating evidence-based practice into decision making in healthcare. Within the literature, goal-setting theory, which was first proposed by Locke and Latham (1990), can be used as a framework for setting goals. This theory is rooted in the development of SMART goals, which are specific, measurable, attainable, relevant, and time-bound (Figure 1.4).

There is no one right way to set a goal, but starting with the possibility that you can meet the goal is good. There's nothing wrong with setting stretch goals to push you beyond your comfort level, but there's nothing more demoralizing than attempting to achieve an unachievable goal (i.e., winning the lottery when I never purchase a ticket). Utilizing statistical techniques with the purpose of developing a statistically sound methodology may make you feel good about your approach, but it may not be the best one. Just because something can be done doesn't mean it should be done. For example, using a statistical technique to set a pneumonia readmission goal may be statistically sound. However, there are many reasons why a patient with pneumonia is readmitted. Any reason for readmission that is not measured will impact the accuracy of the statistical technique being used. These reasons may be beyond your control or the data needed to control for this doesn't

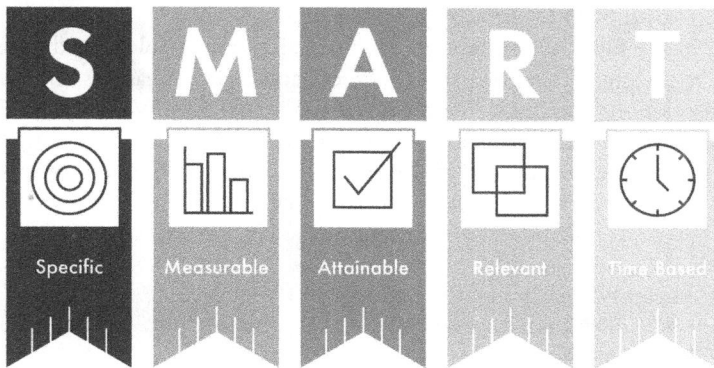

Figure 1.4 SMART Goals.

exist, so using a sound statistical methodology may not make sense from a practical perspective. Sometimes using a percent reduction from a previous baseline measure may be appropriate. Other times developing a SMART goal may be the way to go. The moral of the story is there is no one-size-fits-all approach to developing goals. A percent reduction, statistical model, or goal-setting theory all have their place. What's important is to take a step back and consider all the available information to select the most appropriate goal to drive change.

Conclusion

The Three Pillars of Statistics is our foundation for creating a methodological and statistical approach to drive change. The next step is to build or enhance your current skill set through the introduction of tools and techniques to aid in storytelling with statistics. The next two chapters provide the foundational components to understanding research methodology and statistics. Chapter 2 is a review of research methodology to introduce itse foundational components, such as validity, reliability, scales of measurement, experimental/quasi-experimental design, and survey research. Should you require additional information on a practitioner's focus on research methodology in the real world, a recommended textbook is *Research Methods: Designing and Conducting Research With a Real-World Focus* (Picardi & Masick, 2013).

Chapter 3 reviews statistical concepts analyzed in healthcare with the goal of defining various metrics and introducing the statistical techniques used to derive the metrics. We are firm believers that integrating statistics with research methods is of the utmost importance. In chapter 11 of *Research Methods: Designing and Conducting Research With a Real-World Focus*, Picardi and Masick (2013) focus on integrating statistics with research design to show how they intersect by creating a decision tree to aid in choosing the appropriate statistical test. Should you require further reading on statistical techniques, the series Discovering Statistics

Using… by Andy Field provides a comprehensive view of statistics using various software programs (i.e., SPSS, SAS, and R) (e.g., Field, 2017).

Once you have a baseline understanding of research methodology and statistics, the remaining chapters focus on a variety of healthcare measures/initiatives/ programs. Throughout Chapters 4–9, the approach is the same. While the statistics or methodological design can and likely do vary between chapters, the message will not. Learning how to approach all statistics from a methodological perspective can help you with understanding how the information was derived to help you speak the language of statistics. The structure of the chapters is as follows:

1. Abstract – brief summary of the entire chapter
2. Introduction – introduction/overview of the measures
3. Methodology – methodology of the instrument
4. Results – storytelling with statistics
5. Discussion – behavioral interventions/asking the right analytic question.

The Three Pillars of Statistics ((1) know your numbers; (2) develop behavioral interventions; and (3) set goals to drive change) is the conceptual framework behind the foundation of our toolkit. At the conclusion of this book we aim to develop, refine, or enhance your skill set towards analyzing and presenting metrics with a compelling story. We consider it a success if we teach you at least one new technique to make you more effective in your career, allow you to understand data quicker, or be able to translate numbers into a coherent story backed with the methodological and statistical rigor to drive home the purpose of what you did. Our role isn't to provide clinical guidance as clinical expertise is best left to you! What we can teach you is to take a step back and not jump to conclusions when using data for decision making. Being proactive with analyzing statistics is more effective than being reactive to moving targets. Remember, the pathway to storytelling with data begins with STATISTICS.

Discussion Questions

- Do you believe statistics is an art, a science, or both? Why or why not?
- What are some programs/projects you have implemented using hunches or beliefs, that may have been better suited using statistics?
- How do you see technology playing a role in the future of healthcare analytics?
- What can you do to remain at the cutting edge of change to stay a step ahead of your competitor?
- Think of an intervention you implemented that did not go as planned. What do you think you could have done differently to ensure its success?
- How do you set goals to drive change?
- Should you be proactive or reactive to change?

2 Research Methodology

"Research methodology is like following a recipe; miss a step and the result won't be a cake."

Introduction

The first step in analyzing data is to not jump to conclusions, but rather focus on the methodology of how the statistics are developed. Research methodology is complex and dense, but it is the beginning process of internalizing the analysis for storytelling with statistics. The goal of this chapter is to provide an overview of research methodology in healthcare. Thinking from a methodological perspective will provide a structured step-by-step approach to analyzing any metric. The important concepts within research methodology are reliability (how consistent is data), validity (how accurate is the data), scales of measurement (how metrics are measured), sampling techniques (how data is collected), and research designs (how questions are answered/tested).

Reliability

How does **reliability** relate to healthcare? The simple answer is, it's everywhere. Reliability is the consistency in which a process is implemented, or data is collected. How would you feel if you were making decisions on readmission rates when the data wasn't consistent? How would process improvements or decisions be made with inconsistent data? How would you feel when someone presents data that is inconsistent? On the other hand, anything involving human behavior is likely to have some degree of error associated with it. The point is, consistency in how information is collected is critical for two reasons:

1. Reliability is a necessary, but not sufficient, condition for validity.
2. Reliability is the upper limit to validity.

The first reason means that simply having a reliable or consistent process is not enough for the process to be valid or accurate. Processes can be consistent with a result that is inaccurate. One example is measuring weight with a scale. If the scale is set back 5 lb and only one person knows, then the scale is not valid for anyone who doesn't know this. The scale is deemed reliable, because it is consistently providing a weight every time, but the weight displayed is not accurate. The second reason means that a **validity coefficient** will never be higher than a **reliability coefficient**. In other words, the accuracy of the process is dependent on the consistency of that process. Even though there will likely be some degree of error associated with how a process is measured, it is impossible for an inconsistent process to produce a valid measurement. Questions on the accuracy of a reliable process could be a result of the instrument being used to calculate the measure. For example, the accuracy of measuring a patient's temperature may vary when using multiple thermometers as a result of the calibration of the thermometer.

Knowing that there may be some degree of error in measurements, our goal of presenting data internally within a healthcare organization or externally to the public must be done in a consistent and accurate manner. Any inconsistency within the data collection process may compromise the credibility of results or impact your reputation. With respect to consistency, there are five types of reliability:

1. Test–retest reliability – results on multiple administrations of the same measure to the same person are consistent (i.e., same person taking the same survey twice).
2. Inter/intrarater reliability – ratings between or within raters are similar (i.e., interrater – two different people observing a behavior; intrarater – the same person observing the same behavior twice).
3. Parallel or equivalent forms reliability – developing multiple versions of the same measure (i.e., standardized tests may have multiple versions, but must be equivalent).
4. Split half reliability – a test is divided into two halves and compared for consistency (i.e., a survey divided into even and odd questions which are then compared)
5. Internal consistency/coefficient alpha/Cronbach's alpha – most common technique to compare the consistency of individual items for a single measure (i.e., five items measuring patient experience).

Within healthcare data, two reliability techniques are most widely used. The first is inter/intrarater reliability and the second is coefficient alpha. This isn't to say the other three techniques are not used.

Inter/Intrarater Reliability

From a methodological perspective, there may be times when a hospital/organization develops a data collection tool to collect measures to monitor improvement using either human abstraction or documentation in an electronic medical record (EMR). When this happens, inter/intrarater reliability is used to ensure consistency between abstraction and/or documentation. The purpose of inter/intrarater reliability is to ensure that any monitoring of a metric is done consistently between (**interrater reliability**) different raters or within (**intrarater reliability**) the same rater. Any variability in how others abstract or document data has the potential to compromise the validity or accuracy of the measure being reported. Remember, the accuracy of the decisions relies on a consistent process. Regardless of the reliability technique utilized, data must be consistently reported, so appropriate decisions to drive change are made.

For example, healthcare organizations that abstract severe sepsis/septic shock data for submission to the Centers for Medicare/Medicaid Services (CMS) would want to ensure that all data is captured consistently regardless of the individual abstracting the data or how the information is extracted from the EMR. Under this mandate, CMS released a data definition specification to submit clinical criteria related to severe sepsis/septic shock patients. This document ensures all required variables are accurately defined to eliminate inconsistency. The result of this data could serve multiple purposes. If the end goal is financial incentives, then it's important that data being collected and documented is consistently abstracted or pulled electronically from the medical record. Inconsistent processes could lead to erroneous conclusions, potentially impacting financial reimbursement or the public's perception of a hospital's performance. If the end goal is to develop a risk-adjusted algorithm for severe sepsis/septic shock patients, then inconsistent or inaccurate data collection impacts the accuracy of the risk adjustment.

Regardless of having data specification documents, reliance on human interaction introduces a third variable with subjective interpretation. Having many individuals involved in data collection means there are multiple viewpoints on what definitions mean and how this information is captured across different organizations. Knowing that there is likely to be a degree of error in a measure, eliminating subjectivity in definitions and creating objectivity could increase accurate and consistent measurements. One way of eliminating subjectivity is to develop objective criteria for collecting data (i.e., data definition specification documents). Eliminating gray areas and ensuring a right and a wrong answer is the theoretical method of creating objectivity and eliminating subjectivity. While this may be optimistic, unfortunately it is not easy. Within the realm of collecting data using definitions there will likely always be variability in experience and processes between organizations; Thus, there may always be some degree of error in measurement. The question is, how much variability or error is deemed acceptable?

Internal Consistency/Coefficient Alpha/Cronbach's Alpha

The other type of reliability within healthcare has many names: **internal consistency, coefficient alpha,** or **Cronbach's alpha reliability**. Regardless of how you refer to it, this reliability technique is used when multiple items are created to measure one variable. Traditionally, asking one question to someone may be quick and easy; most constructs (i.e., patient experience) are multi-faceted. Simply asking a patient to rate their experience in the hospital or physician's office could be defined multiple ways. One question would be unable to capture the depth of a patient's experience. Internal consistency reliability examines the relationship between all items measuring patient experience and determines if they actually *do* measure patient experience. Internal consistency determines the relationship between multiple items and ranges from 0 to 1 where a value closer to 1 indicates higher reliability. A general acceptable level of internal consistency is greater than or equal to 0.7 (Cronbach, 1951).

Patient experience measures are an example of internal consistency. Patient experience is measured by Hospital Consumer Assessment of Healthcare Providers and Systems (HCAHPS) using 32 questions to assess 11 different domains. One particular domain on the HCAHPS survey is pain management. This domain consists of multiple questions addressing various aspects of pain management. In this case, the purpose of internal consistency is that all questions measuring pain management actually measure that domain with an internal consistency of greater than or equal to 0.7. Should the internal consistency be less than 0.7, then the content of the individual items must be addressed. If the individual items for pain management include a question on likelihood to recommend, then the internal consistency would be lower. Pain management questions are designed to assess patient perceptions surrounding their level of pain or how well their level of pain is being controlled. This differs from likelihood to recommend, which would be asking patients whether or not they would recommend this organization to others. As a result, the questions asking about pain management are unrelated to likelihood to recommend and therefore, only questions measuring the measure of interest should be included. The analysis of these individual items is known as the field of psychometrics, which is devoted towards advancing quantitative measures of variables.

Validity

Now that we have addressed the consistency of a process, we are going to transition to the accuracy that process produces. If a measure cannot consistently be collected, then how can a result be accurate? Reliability is the consistency of measuring a metric and is a necessary, but not sufficient, condition for **validity**. This means a valid metric must also be reliable, because there will never be a situation where a metric is valid and not reliable. Take a step back and think about the following two questions to differentiate the purpose of reliability and validity:

1. Is my data collection tool consistently doing what it is supposed to do?
2. Are the results I'm getting from my data collection tool accurate?

Pay close attention to the nuances between those two questions. The first is asking about the purpose of what the tool is supposed to be doing or the process to consistently collect data. The process of how data is collected is not directly related to the accuracy of the data collected. The second is asking about the accuracy of the results from the tool and not the process used to collect the data. The accuracy of conclusions is defined by four main types of validity:

1. External validity
2. Construct validity
3. Statistical conclusion validity
4. Internal validity.

All four types of validity are critically important, but two that stand out from a methodological perspective is how metrics are defined (i.e., construct validity) and if these results apply to other samples or population (i.e., external validity). The accuracy of the statistical technique (i.e., statistical conclusion validity) and any other explanation (i.e, internal validity) for how the data is being collected are other aspects of validity that impact results. External and construct validity are critical for creating and explaining metrics. Internal and statistical conclusion validity are critical in ensuring no other explanation can describe the results and choosing the right statistic. Readers interested in a further review of validity and reliability are advised to consult a research methodology textbook.

External Validity

Whenever evaluating any metric or research study, concerns with the **generalizability** of the results are often critiqued. In other words, will the results found from this metric or research study be the same with other participants, settings, outcomes, and/or treatments? These four variations in results are referred to as threats to external validity. To think of them in an applied way, consider framing the threats with questions:

1. Participants – Would these metrics be the same with a different sample?
2. Settings – Would the metrics from one hospital generalize to another? Or would the metrics generalize from one patient population to another?
3. Outcome – Would the results be the same if another variable was measured?
4. Treatment – Would the results be the same if the intervention was modified or changed?

To relate this to healthcare, think of a **risk-adjusted measure** of mortality used to compare a hospital's performance to another hospital. CMS Hospital Compare data is publicly available and uses risk-adjusted metrics analyzed over a 3-year timeframe. From an external validity perspective, alternative explanations for how this information generalizes to any one of the four external validity threats exist. The following examples are critiques of external validity with risk-adjusted measures.

1. Participants – This data is based on Medicare patients only, so results may not generalize to other non-Medicare patient populations.
2. Settings – Could this model be applied to patients who arrive at the emergency department and are not admitted?
3. Outcomes – Could this risk-adjusted mortality model be used to risk adjust readmission measures?
4. Treatments – How do modifications/changes to treatment of patients or documentation of treatments impact the risk adjustment model?

The statistical rigor put into the development of these models is sound from both a statistical and research methodological perspective. Thinking methodologically about any statistic helps to understand the implications of the results. Remember, don't be defensive; be proactive. Rationalizing or discrediting statistics presented doesn't fix or change the results.

Construct Validity

Other types of critiques revolve around the numerator and denominator of a variable. **Construct validity** is related to the **operationalization** or how the measure is being defined. Knowing the numerator, denominator, inclusion, and exclusion criteria for every metric is key to knowing how performance is being assessed. Any question related to how a metric is defined would be considered a threat to construct validity. Shadish, Cook, and Campbell (2002) identify construct validity as being important for three reasons:

1. Constructs connect the information used within experiments to theory.
2. Constructs have specific labels that carry implications.
3. Constructs are continually created and defended.

When developing constructs to accurately measure and engage in change, it's critically important these metrics are defined thoroughly. When we implement change, we have an idea or theory behind what the results will be or how we can go about improving a phenomenon of interest. These constructs have been defined in many ways with specific implications. Looking at the construct "readmission" you can find many different definitions around this metric. CMS has its own definition that carries financial penalties/incentives, clinicians may have a different variation to the definition aimed at how to clinically reduce readmissions, definitions may vary between a physician office, hospital, emergency department, or peer-reviewed published literature. The point is that every definition is correct in its own way and has very specific labels that come with the construct. These definitions could be partly responsible for why new construct definitions are created and existing ones defended.

Defining constructs is not easy. Try and ask multiple people how they would define customer satisfaction and see if they are all defined and measured the same. Within construct validity, there are 14 threats that compromise how a metric is defined, which is grouped into three categories: definition of variables, researcher/participant issues, and implementation of design (Picardi & Masick, 2013). Questioning the accuracy of the definition occurs at multiple points in the process, whether it's determining an initial definition for a measured construct to how others may perceive this definition during the development phase and through the data collection phase. Regardless of where the issues are with a definition, the purpose of defining a metric is to ensure it measures what it's intended to measure. Any gray area in the definition could lead to misinterpretation or incorrect measurements. This lack of clarity is the most problematic and is referred to as **inadequate explication of constructs** (Brutus, Gill, & Duniewicz, 2010).

For example, referring to the construct of patient satisfaction, there are multiple vendors with varying definitions for how patient satisfaction is measured. Is patient satisfaction defined as how satisfied a patient is with their hospital experience? Communication with healthcare professionals? Time spent in the emergency department? Cleanliness of the hospital? Quality of the food? Time spent in a physician's office? And so forth. All of these definitions may reflect aspects of patient satisfaction but implementing change to improve this metric requires an understanding of how it is measured. What if a definition for patient satisfaction was the "quality of the information provided to you by a healthcare professional regarding your treatment plan?" Is this a clear question that every patient will interpret the same?

Let's break that definition apart. What does quality mean? Each person may internalize what quality means to them. What kind of information? Throughout a hospital stay there is a lot of information that a patient may need, ranging from clinical variables (i.e., important labs, radiology tests, etc.) to non-clinical variables (i.e., when are the meals being delivered or where is the bathroom, etc.). The end of the statement attempts to clarify the information by specifying a treatment plan. However, is the treatment plan based on what is being done in the hospital or what to do after the hospitalization? Any variation in how a patient interprets this is a threat to the validity of the metric and will result in a degree of error when combining data with other patients. It is virtually impossible to assess every aspect of patient satisfaction. Instead what happens is researchers study these constructs and analyze the internal consistency reliability to make sure the created items measure patient satisfaction. Creating improvement initiatives on what you *think* is being measured vs. what is *actually* measured will not result in change.

Statistical Conclusion and Internal Validity

The last two types of validity are discussed at a high level. Readers interested in a more thorough explanation are encouraged to consult a research methods book. Both are related to alternative explanations for how results are interpreted. Think of internal validity as someone skeptical of all results. This person can think of every reason for why the results are wrong. For example, think of an intervention aimed to reduce heart failure readmissions by initiating weekly phone calls post hospital discharge. Before even looking at the results, any explanation for why a patient is readmitted or not is a threat to internal validity. Some reasons may be: medication issues, lack of social support, discharge planning, or any reason unrelated to heart failure, etc. The list of reasons is larger than that, but the point is any alternative explanation beyond the phone call intervention could explain why the patient was readmitted, which threatens the accuracy of the results. Questioning and being skeptical about data help to avoid any alternative explanation that compromises the accuracy of the results. It also helps to make you proactive with anticipating potential criticism of results.

Statistical conclusion validity is mainly related to using the correct statistical analysis for the collected data. Statistical software is extremely helpful to do complex analyses, but it's important to know what you are doing and why. Programs are used to analyze data. They don't know if you have adequate power. You can examine the results of the analysis to see if you have adequate power, but no one is telling you not to conduct the analysis. You control the analysis, so a program would allow you to quantitatively analyze a value of gender that is entered as a 1 for female and 2 for male. You would be able to calculate a mean and standard deviation. The point is that statistical programs are only as smart as the individual doing the analysis. Statistical conclusion validity is meant to ensure that the right statistics are chosen. Part of this battle begins with an understanding of how data is measured.

Scales of Measurement

With the discussion of metrics and the importance of consistent and accurate measures, the next phase of metric development is understanding how to measure them. There are four ways a metric is measured, which is referred to as scales of measurement. Scales of measurement are hierarchical with each scale having its own unique properties, but scales above on the hierarchy can be transformed to any scale appearing below it on the hierarchy. The four scales are categorized as **qualitative scales of measurement** and **quantitative scales of measurement** where the selected scale of measurement will dictate the type of statistical analysis. Qualitative scales of measurement are nominal and ordinal scales and quantitative scales of measurement are interval and ratio.

Qualitative Scales of Measurement

Nominal Scale

The nominal scale is the lowest on this hierarchy. A nominal scale's purpose is assigning arbitrary numbers to name a variable. For example, a nominal scale is used for gender to assign a value of 1 to females and 2 to males. These numbers have no quantitative properties and only serve as a naming convention to analyze data. Nominal data is converted to percentages when telling a story (i.e., there were 43% males and 57% females).

Ordinal Scale

The purpose of an ordinal scale is to rank order items to determine what value is larger or smaller than another. This could involve rank ordering responses on a survey or the order that patients arrive in an emergency department. The only information an ordinal scale has is knowing which patient came into the emergency department first, second, third, etc., without knowing how much time has elapsed between the first and second patient. Ordinal data does not require equal intervals between rank orders, so the first patient could have come in at 9:00am, the second at 9:03am, and the third at 12:00pm. They would be labeled as 1, 2, and 3.

Box 2.1 Nominal Data – The Case of Arbitrary vs. Non-Arbitrary Data

There's a twist with nominal data and it involves questioning the word arbitrary. Think about mortality or readmission data. We assign a value of 1 or 0 to mortality and readmission, so patients who expire or are readmitted are assigned a value of 1 and patients who are alive or not readmitted are assigned a value of 0. This would be a classic case of nominal data in the way that gender could be assigned as a 1 or 2, or even a 0 or 1, to indicate females or males. The caveat with nominal data having quantitative properties (i.e., mean or standard deviation) is when the assigned value carries meaning, which means the assigned value is not arbitrary. With binary data (1 and 0) in the case of mortality or readmission, the value of 1 indicates the presence of an event and a 0 indicates the absence of an event. While it appears nominal in nature, the assigned value carries meaning. For example, if you are calculating mortality rates for 100 people and you use 1 to indicate expired and 0 to indicate alive, then 20 expirations would be equivalent to 20%. If no patients died, then this would be a true 0 where there are no deaths. Likewise, if there were 5 expirations one month and the next month there were 10, then you could state that twice as many patients expired this month compared to last. Binary data, where assigned values have meaning, can be treated quantitatively as ratio scales.

Quantitative Scales of Measurement

Interval Scale

Interval scales enhance the ordinal scale properties with equal intervals between each data point, but no true 0 (an absence/non-existence of whatever is measured). The most common and widely used interval scale is a Likert-type scale that consists of a 5–7-point rating scale; for example, a 1–5-point Likert-type satisfaction scale where 1 is "completely dissatisfied" and 5 is "completely satisfied." Quantitative statistics, such as means and standard deviations, can be calculated from interval scales (refer to Chapter 3 for statistical terminology). Another type of interval scale is temperature measured in degrees Fahrenheit. There is an equal interval between degrees, but there is no true 0. This means that 0 degrees Fahrenheit does not indicate a complete absence of temperature.

While Likert-type scales are used to quantify behaviors, it is important to note that various disciplines deal with Likert-type scales differently. Within the realm of psychology, Likert-type scales are considered interval scales. Biostatistics may refer to these scales as ordinal, because 5 is larger than 4, but the interval between 1 and 2 may not be the same as that from 4 to 5. With that said, interval scales add significant value statistically because of the ability to quantitatively analyze them.

Ratio Scales

The final scale is a ratio scale. A ratio scale has all the properties of every other scale, but the difference in this scale is the presence of a true 0. This means that every interval on a given scale can be quantified. For example, age is a ratio scale. One could have a philosophical argument that an age of 0 doesn't necessarily mean that something isn't alive. The counterargument is that a measure is always a ratio scale if a statement can be made that one value is two or three times another value. With age, someone who is 40 years old is twice as old as a 20-year-old. This doesn't apply to interval scales, because a rating of 4 on a satisfaction scale doesn't mean that this person is twice as satisfied as a rating of 2.

Scales of Measurement Discussion

Deciding what scale to measure variables is a complicated decision, but it's one that cannot be taken lightly. The hierarchical nature of scales of measurement means that every scale above the lowest in the hierarchy can be transformed into a lower scale. One of Kevin's colleagues, Larry Lutsky, discussed this issue before and stressed the importance of measuring the variable at the scale of measurement it was designed to be. For example, age is measured as a ratio scale, but can be transformed to age categories, such as interval (e.g., 0–9, 10–19, 20–29, 30–39, etc.), ordinal (e.g., <18, 18–65, 65+), or nominal (baby, toddler, youth, teenagers, adults, elderly, etc.). This is problematic for two reasons: (1) changing the scale of measurement changes the statistical analyses that can be conducted; and (2) nominal and ordinal scales of measurement are qualitative; interval and ratio scales of measurement are quantitative. Calculating a mean and standard deviation is lost when transforming metrics to a qualitative scale. Statistical techniques exist to estimate the mean when an age range is provided, but it's only an estimate that will have some degree of error (i.e., threat to validity) associated with it.

Sampling Techniques

The process of thinking methodologically starts with the consistency (reliability) and accuracy (validity) when analyzing data and how data is measured (scales of measurement). The next step involves understanding how data is collected (**sampling**). Whether conducting research or evaluating survey results, understanding how the sample was selected is necessary. There are two main sampling techniques:

1. Probability sampling
2. Non-probability sampling.

Collecting data from the entire population is costly and time consuming, which may be unnecessary; this is the advantage of sampling. Sampling is done to select a statistically valid sample from the population to generalize results from the sample back to the population. This generalization of results is the main premise of external validity.

Probability Sampling

Probability is the chance of something occurring that ranges between 0 and 1, with 0 being no chance of something happening and 1 being 100% chance of something happening. This sampling technique ensures that everyone in the population has an equal chance of being selected to be in the sample, thus ensuring the random sample is representative of the population. The one caveat to probability sampling is that the entire population must be known. If you do not know or have access to the entire population of interest, then you cannot conduct a probability sampling technique. Within probability sampling techniques, there are three different options: **simple random sampling, stratified sampling,** and **cluster sampling**.

- Simple random sampling – using a random number generator, such as the Rand() function in Microsoft Excel, to randomly select your sample.
- Stratified sampling – dividing the population into subgroups, or strata (i.e., nurses and physicians, or administrative, clinical, and non-clinical), and selecting a random sample.
- Cluster sampling – dividing the population into groups or clusters by geographical location, for example, and then selecting a random sample.

Non-probability Sampling

When it is not possible to know or have access to the entire population, then non-probability sampling is used. Non-probability means a sample selected is not based on chance, so the sample may not be representative of the population, which impacts on external validity or the generalization of results. Within non-probability sampling there are four options: convenience sampling, snowball sampling, quota sampling, and purposive sampling.

- **Convenience sampling** – selecting the sample based on who you have access to
- **Snowball sampling** – selecting a sample where current participants are used to obtain additional participants (i.e., using a participant with a rare condition to find others with the same condition)
- **Quota sampling** – similar to stratified sampling where a population is divided into subgroups. The difference is being told how many individuals based on a criterion of interest to collect data from
- **Purposive sampling** – selecting a sample based on specific criterion that is relevant to the research question of interest (i.e., selecting females for a study on women's health)

In the end, choosing a probability or non-probability sampling technique is not as critical as knowing whether or not it's possible to access the entire population. This impacts how results are generalized to other people, settings, outcomes, or treatments (i.e., external validity) and can impact the conclusions.

Research Methodology

When analyzing metrics (scales of measurement), the data must be collected (sampling) consistently (reliability) to provide accurate (validity) results for decision making, goal setting, and driving change. The entire process of analyzing data starts by thinking methodologically. Research methodology is complex, but it's the technique that creates structure around collecting and analyzing data. Too often we believe we know what we're doing or we learned that concept before, but do you *really* know your numbers when it comes to statistics? What goes into creating a number or metric is more complex than what it represents and taking action from data is not always straightforward. Have you ever wondered about the process of how we learn? To begin, there are two categories: **basic research** and **applied research**. Basic research is used to understand a process without creating new knowledge. Applied research is used to solve problems by predicting a phenomenon of interest or a reaction to a situation. Within healthcare, the process of storytelling using statistics begins with analyzing a dataset to understand a process. Therefore, basic research must be used to understand a process prior to using applied research to solve the problem.

From a big picture perspective, the start of any initiative begins with having input into the concept. This input provides the process to accomplish the intervention with a result of improving an outcome of interest. How do these concepts fit together to accomplish the goal of telling a story? Process or performance improvement is a journey, so don't expect change to happen overnight. Take the time to think methodologically and focus on the journey, not the destination or end result. Remember, whenever evaluating analytics or data to tell a story, the most critical piece is understanding the methodology behind the metrics presented.

Within research methodology, there are four main categories: (1) non-experimental; (2) quasi-experimental; (3) experimental; and (4) survey research (survey research is its own category because it can be any research category). Each research category has advantages and disadvantages, but no one design is better than the other. Approach every situation by thinking methodologically to determine an appropriate research design to answer your question.

Non-experimental Research

Non-experimental research is the precursor to conducting research and doesn't imply any cause-and-effect relationship. The most common type of non-experimental research is a **correlational design**. With correlations the key phrase to remember is "correlation does not mean causation." For example, researchers have examined relationships between the Agency for Healthcare Research and Quality (AHRQ) patient safety survey, patient outcomes, and patient satisfaction (DiCuccio, 2015; Junewicz & Youngner, 2015; Manary, Boulding, Staelin, and Glickman, 2013; Mardon, Khanna, Sorra, Dyer, & Famolaro, 2010; Trzeciak, Gaughan, Bosire, & Mazzarelli, 2016; Weaver, Lubomski, Wilson, Pfoh, Martinez, & Dy, 2013). They do not imply any of these variables cause another, but rather that they all share some kind of relationship. A correlational design will tell you exactly what kind of relationship they share.

Quasi-experimental Research

Quasi-experimental research examines cause-and-effect relationships between independent variables (variable manipulated) and dependent variables (variable measured) to state that the manipulation affected the measurement. Quasi-experimental design lacks **random assignment**, so selected participants are not assigned to groups randomly or by chance. This means groups may differ before the start of the experiment, which is a common threat to internal validity. Lack of random assignment can be overcome by implementing design features (i.e., pre-test and post-test or control groups) to reduce threats to internal validity or alternative explanations that compromise the accuracy of the results.

Experimental Research

Experimental research has the same characteristics and features of quasi-experimental design, but utilizes random assignment to create different groups based on chance. Having random assignment ensures randomly created groups and alleviates some threats to internal validity. Experimental research is viewed as the gold standard to conducting research and is used in clinical trials, but other research designs are equally effective. The compromise is that experimental research may minimize threats to internal validity through random assignment, but highly controlled research may not have external validity in practice.

Survey Research

Survey research is different from the rest, as it can be experimental, non-experimental, or quasi-experimental in design. For instance, results from surveys can capture the entire population or a sample of the population. Survey research is common within healthcare. HCAHPS is a well-known patient satisfaction survey administered to patients. Many healthcare professionals may choose to do survey research because the belief is that it is easier to create a survey than develop an experimental or quasi-experimental research study. Designing a survey takes skill and knowledge to execute effectively. Creating your own survey questions may not be valid or reliable, so finding and using a validated survey are more effective than creating one.

Research Methodology Discussion

All research designs have their own advantages and disadvantages and no one design is better than another. To think methodologically, focusing on specific questions can guide the decision making. As a healthcare professional, how much time do you spend gathering information from a patient prior to diagnosing him/her? Now how much time do you spend understanding the statistics you're analyzing?

We assume the time spent diagnosing a patient is longer than the time spent making decisions when looking at a metric. Why? Are there no clear techniques on what to look for with data as there are with diagnosing patients? You may have different techniques or tools to solicit necessary information for a diagnosis, but may not have any techniques for analyzing data. This process of collecting information is done following a process or methodologically. Having a methodological approach to gathering information is an effective way to ensure all the required information is systematically collected prior to making decisions. To enhance a methodological approach to data, we created the DEFINE tool:

- D: Denominator – what is your population of interest?
- E: Exclusion criteria – are there any variables that are going to be excluded from your population, sample, or statistic?
- F: Factor – what is it multiplied by? How is your statistic calculated?
- I: Inclusion criteria – are there any variables that are going to be included from your population, sample, or statistic?
- N: Numerator – what part of your population is eligible to be part of the event?
- E: Evaluate all the information to ensure there are no holes in the definition.

Understanding the data analysis is as important as gathering information from a patient to provide a diagnosis. Decisions are driven by data, so devote the required time to methodologically collect the information and understand the metrics. The DEFINE tool encourages methodological thinking and structures necessary questions to understand how a metric is defined. Here's an example using DEFINE for understanding severe sepsis mortality (Table 2.1).

Research designs focus on basic research to understand a process without creating new knowledge. Applied research focuses on solving problems. While the research designs discussed can focus on depending on how a study is set up, two applied research techniques utilized within healthcare are root cause analysis (RCA) and plan–do–study–act (PDSA). An RCA approach uses an interdisciplinary team to get to the root cause of a problem through continually asking the question "Why?" until no more answers can be provided. The end result is the root cause of why an issue occurred. PDSA is a cyclical approach similar to the scientific method. It is meant to answer a question by going through a process or methodology. The plan phase involves an introduction to addressing a problem by carefully planning what to accomplish. The do phase involves developing a sound methodology to answer the question posed in the plan phase. The study phase is where data is collected and analyzed. The final act phase is where the results are put into action. A variation of this methodology was introduced by the Institute for Healthcare Improvement (IHI) and is referred to as rapid PDSA cycles. Within rapid PDSA cycles change occurs quickly by implementing a process change followed by studying the impact of the change with a handful of observations before making another change. This rapid PDSA cycle is effective to address continuous improvement and test small changes quickly. For example, testing process changes for treating severe sepsis/septic shock patients could involve studying a

Table 2.1 DEFINE tool example

DEFINE tool	Question	Answer
D – Denominator	Who is included in your patient population?	Any patient >18 years old who was diagnosed with severe sepsis
E – Exclusion criteria	Are there any patients excluded from your population?	Patients < 18 years old and hospice patients are excluded
F – Factor	How is your metric calculated?	Numerator/denominator multiplied by 100 to convert to a percentage
I – Inclusion criteria	What patient population is included?	A secondary diagnosis code of severe sepsis
N – Numerator	What is your numerator? Or what patient population has the opportunity to be included in the calculation?	Any patient who dies in the hospital diagnosed with severe sepsis
E – Evaluate	Have you included all possible information or are there any holes in your methodology?	What is the rationale for excluding patients < 18 years old? Is a severe sepsis diagnosis done with primary and secondary codes? Could diagnosis-related groups (DRGs) be used?

change in the process of collecting blood cultures for 5 patients, then moving to another process change for 5 different patients until a desired effective process is achieved and replicated.

In conclusion, the focus of the current chapter was to provide an overview of various components of research methodology to approach performance/quality improvement in a methodological way. The next chapter focuses on statistical concepts within healthcare to learn how to interpret data in healthcare and analyze numbers methodologically.

Discussion Questions

- What would you do if you were listening to a presentation and you knew the data presented was not consistent?
- Do you agree that a reliable process may not be valid, but a valid process will always be reliable?
  Can you think of an example where a process is valid, but not reliable?
- Knowing any type of human interaction in a process could result in an error in measurement, what could you do to eliminate inconsistent processes?
- Come up with your own definition for a metric of interest and see if others agree with the accuracy of your metric.
- A ratio scale of measure can be converted to any of the other three scales (nominal, ordinal or interval). Compare and contrast the advantages/disadvantages of doing that.

- Why do you think it matters how data is sampled?
- Not knowing or having access to the entire population means you can't do a probability sampling technique. What are some populations of interest that you do have access to?
- Your colleague discounts the effectiveness of non-probability sampling techniques since there's no way of knowing if the sample represents the population. How would you convince your colleague that non-probability sampling techniques are helpful?
- Can you create a research study using the same variables that could fit all four categories (non-experimental, quasi-experimental, experimental, and survey research)?
- How will the DEFINE tool help you with understanding metrics?

3   Statistics

"Expecting statistics to provide the answer means you asked the wrong question."

Introduction

Some may believe that statistics are the answer when in fact statistics are the questions. There may be some pre-conceived notions that a statistical analysis can provide the answers. Yes, they do provide an answer, but statistics should generate more questions. Are you the type of person who shudders at the word "statistics"? Do you feel anxiety when explaining statistics? Do you feel overwhelmed with analyzing metrics, because you don't truly understand them? Does translating numbers into a story seem like a mystery? Feeling stressed with statistics is common. We can alleviate this stress by providing techniques on simple solutions for approaching a statistical problem. This is done by building a relationship between statistics and research methodology to systematically break down the numbers into meaningful pieces. Analyzing metrics without understanding the methodology behind them leads to incorrect results. Any decision made on how to collect data impacts the statistical analysis. Focusing on the results without understanding the methodology is a mistake.

A conceptual understanding of statistics aids in having the ability to apply that knowledge to maximize statistical interpretation. When learning statistics, students often ask, "so how does this work in the real world?" Focusing on teaching statistical theory without an applied understanding is not effective in translating concepts into practice or seeing students have that "aha" moment. Through teaching statistics with an applied focus, it is evident how often statistics are encountered in our daily lives. Therefore, it is our goal to teach anyone to critically think about and evaluate numbers to tell a story using statistics. Another example to illustrate the integration of research methodology and statistics is using readmission rates. Readmission rates are interpreted as rates or percentages. When thinking about interpreting the metric as a rate or percentage, the calculation and story are the same. The metric is calculated as the sum of all readmissions divided by the sum of the total discharges with the result multiplied by 100. For example, 200 readmissions divided by 1,000 discharges equals 0.2. Multiplying this value by 100 yields 20. The rate interpretation is 20 patients per 100 discharges and the percentage interpretation is that 20% of discharges are readmitted. Regardless of whether or not a rate is interpreted as a percentage or per 100 discharges, the result is the same.

Thinking methodologically started with an understanding of how this 20% readmission rate is calculated. What is the scale of measurement? Is it a nominal, ordinal, interval, or ratio scale? Readmission rates range from 0 to 100%, with 0% being no readmissions and where a rate of 40% is twice as high as a rate of 20%, so is it a ratio scale? By these standards it would be ratio, but this is wrong. Think back to Chapter 2 and what would Larry say? He would say to focus on the unit of measurement, so in this case the unit of measure is whether or not a patient was readmitted, which would be coded as 1 for a readmit and 0 for not being readmitted. This is equivalent to a nominal scale. Are you surprised? Did you rush to make a decision or actually think about it? Step back and think methodologically about this example. Readmission rates are calculated by the total number of readmitted patients divided by all discharged patients. There may be some inclusion and exclusion criteria to define readmissions, but this is not important for determining the scale of measurement. Every patient has two options: they are either readmitted or not readmitted. This classification is categorical. A value of 1 is assigned to a readmitted patient and 0 for a patient not readmitted. Whenever a value is assigned to a word, then this is a nominal scale. These nominal scale values are then aggregated and converted to percentages with the purpose of telling a story about readmissions. A percentage controls for fluctuations in monthly volume and adds context to the story. For example, Table 3.1 provides 6 months of readmissions. Focusing only on the total number of readmissions indicates that there are 100 readmissions each month, with no ability to determine if the number of monthly readmissions is increasing or decreasing. Converting nominal data to a percentage paints a different picture and enhances the story to ask different questions (i.e., what may have happened in March? Or why is the readmission rate decreasing?)

Understanding the statistical methodology behind a metric is the key to understanding statistics. A methodology or process transcends all of statistics. Knowing how to break down the information into meaningful pieces aids in a better understanding of how to interpret metrics. With that said, the following sections provide an overview of statistics in healthcare. Future chapters utilize these statistical concepts to aid in storytelling with statistics.

Table 3.1 Monthly readmissions

Month	Readmissions	Discharges	Percentage
January	100	567	17.6%
February	100	892	11.2%
March	100	421	23.8%
April	100	534	18.7%
May	100	1031	9.7%
June	100	993	10.1%

Alpha and Type I Error

Alpha, beta, and **power** are critical when conducting research and understanding if something is significant, which is called statistical significance (i.e., a *p* value). The significance level is known as **alpha, alpha level, *p* value, or α** and ranges from 0 to 1. *p* Values are a measure of probability or chance of something happening. Common acceptable *p* values for indicating statistical significance are 0.05, 0.01, and 0.001. The interpretation of *p* values less than one of those three values means statistical significance. Any value above 0.05 indicates no statistical significance. *p* Values can be interpreted as percentages, so a 0.05, 0.01, or 0.001 *p* value converts to 5%, 1%, or 0.1%, respectively. This percentage of alpha is equivalent to the chance of making a **type I error** or saying something is not significant when it is.

Beta and Type II Error

Beta or β cannot be set, but can be influenced using methodological design (i.e., sample size). Beta is also based on probability and ranges from 0 to 1. These values can be converted to percentages, but there is no set beta level to determine statistical significance. The beta value is interpreted as the probability or percent chance of making a **type II error.** A beta value of 0.2 would indicate a 20% chance of making a type II error or saying something is significant when it is not.

Power

Although the level of beta cannot be set, it can be influenced by power. The formula for power is derived by 1 − beta (β), therefore beta is intertwined with power and power is something that can be controlled by you. Beta is the chance of not finding statistical significance and statistical **power** is the chance of finding statistical significance. Power ranges from 0 to 1 and can be converted to a percentage. The relationship between power and beta is based on the formula, so they always add up to 100%. A general rule of thumb is having a power of 0.8 is acceptable, which means that there is a 0.2 or 20% chance of making a type II error.

Having a high power indicates a greater chance of statistical significance with a lower chance of making a type II error, so we could be saying something is significant when it may not be. This power–beta relationship can be influenced by sample size. The larger the sample size, the higher the power (Table 3.2). We may often think that the best path to analyzing data is to have as much data as possible. However, collecting data to achieve a high power is not desirable as it can lead to erroneous conclusions, which would be finding trivial differences that are not clinically meaningful. It is highly recommended to conduct a power analysis to determine an adequate and appropriate sample size to find statistical significance before data is collected. In other words, collect the right amount of data to find out if your results are significant. On the other hand, a low power means a higher chance of a type II error. For further review and discussion of statistical power, readers should consult the *Statistical Power Analysis for the Behavioral Sciences* textbook by Cohen (1988).

Table 3.2 The power phenomenon

n Size	p Value
25	0.59
50	0.44
100	0.28
150	0.18
250	0.09
300	0.06
350	0.04

In referencing Table 3.2 and the relationship between sample size and alpha, let's look at an example. The example is comparing two groups based on an intertevention to reduce length of stay. An a priori power analysis with a medium effect (i.e., strength of the acceptable sample size to determine significance would be 102. Group 1 is the treatment group and group 2 is the control group. The actual intervention is irrelevant for this illustration. The mean and standard deviation remain constant and the only change is based on increasing the sample size. An independent sample *t*-test is used to test the differences between a group 1 mean of 5.1 with a standard deviation of 1.3 and group 2 is a mean of 5.3 with a standard deviation of 1.3. Collecting data using the a priori power analysis

---

Box 3.1 Wrong Decisions Happen

When analyzing statistics or conducting research, there are three important points: (1) decreased type I error; (2) decreased type II error; and (3) appropriate power. You can't have it all. Being right 100% of the time is not likely, so making a statistical error is possible; if not inevitable at some point. Type I errors occur when a significant relationship exists that really doesn't or you say something works when it doesn't. Type II errors occur when no significant relationship exists that really does or you say something doesn't work when it does. As a healthcare professional, would you rather be making a type I or type II error? In practice, a type I error would be saying something (i.e., surgery, medication, intervention, etc.) is effective when it really is not. A type II error is saying something doesn't work when it really does. Would you want to be told that a medication is helping when it really isn't or that the medication doesn't work when it really does? It's the whole tradeoff of where to be wrong. Within the literature, the *p* value is used to determine statistical significant. Any *p* value less than 0.05, 0.01, or 0.001 is statistically significant. This indicates that being wrong 5%, 1%, or 0.1% is the acceptable benchmark for determining significance. While the focus may be more on type I errors, type II errors can't be ignored.

resulting in a sample of 102 would result in a non-significant value. However, if a researcher decides to collect as much data as possible, then by the time there is a sample of 350 or greater the difference between group 1 and 2 becomes statistically significant. This highlights the importance of only collecting the minimally acceptable sample to determine statistical significance.

Statistical Significance vs. Clinical Significance

Statistical significance may be viewed as the gold standard for determining whether or not a relationship exists. Relying on only statistical significance and not considering other factors can be problematic. There are two pieces for beginning to tell a story with statistics: understanding the statistical significance of the results and knowing the clinical significance of those results. It is possible that statistical significance can be found between a mortality rate of 3.4% and 3.7%. A large enough sample size can result in a high enough power to detect significance. Statistical significance, while important, is not the only answer. Results from statistical tests may be statistically significant but not clinically significant, or vice versa. Relying solely on statistical significance may lead to the wrong conclusion. This is where it's crucial to consider if the results have any clinical meaningfulness. A desire to only have statistically significant results could end up being clinically meaningless. Likewise, the desire for clinical significance could end up being statistically insignificant. There is much to learn from both scenarios, so continue to leverage the available tools to critically think about the situation.

Descriptive/Inferential Statistics

There are two categories of statistics: (1) **descriptive** and (2) **inferential** statistics. Put simply, descriptive statistics are designed to *describe* or summarize data. Inferential statistics are designed to *infer* or deduce information from data. Whether or not the analysis involves descriptive or inferential statistics, the following concepts apply to both, with the only difference being the interpretation.

Measures of Central Tendency

Measures of central tendency enhance the interpretation of the results using the **mean, median,** and **mode.** The mean is the average and most widely reported measure of central tendency. There are multiple types of means available given certain characteristics of the data being analyzed. In generic terms, calculating the mean involves adding all values and dividing by the total count. For example, a mortality rate is calculated by adding the total number of deaths and dividing by the total number of patients discharged; this number is then converted to a percentage. This calculation is referred to as an arithmetic mean with normally distributed data. Outliers or extreme values and skewed data have an impact on the arithmetic mean, so geometric and trimmed means are alternatives that account for extreme values (i.e., calculating length of stay).

Table 3.3 The influence of outliers

5 Patients' length of stay	Arithmetic mean	Median	Standard deviation	Geometric mean
3, 5, 6, 9, 120	28.6	6	51.14	9.9
3, 5, 6, 9, 11	6.8	6	3.19	6.2

The median is the number in the middle of a data set. The median is useful when data is **skewed** (not normally distributed). **Outliers** can impact the normal distribution and have more of an influence on the mean than median. For example, a patient with a length of stay (LOS) of 120 days impacts the mean and skews the data, which makes the arithmetic mean not ideal. As an alternative, the median or **geometric mean** is used in place of the arithmetic mean. In Table 3.3, the impact of the 120-day LOS is shown with the various calculations. The five patients in the first example have an outlier (120-day LOS) that results in an arithmetic mean of 28.6 days, a median of 6, and a geometric mean of 9.9 with a standard deviation of 51.14 days. The second example does not have an outlier and the arithmetic mean is 6.8 days, median is 6 days, and geometric mean is 6.2 days with a standard deviation of 3.19 days. With skewed data, the median or geometric mean may better represent the dataset instead of the arithmetic mean.

The final measure of central tendency is the mode, which is the value(s) that appear(s) most often. A dataset with more than one mode is bimodal (two modes), trimodal (three modes), or multimodal (four or more modes).

Measures of Dispersion

Measures of dispersion are used to examine variability within a dataset using **range, variance, standard deviation,** or **interquartile range**. The inclusion of multiple statistics, such as measures of central tendency and dispersion, enhances the story. The range is a crude measure of variability calculated by subtracting the largest and smallest value in a dataset. Both variance and standard deviation are measures of dispersion around the mean, but their interpretations are vastly different. Variance has multiple definitions depending on how it is being referenced. Two common references involve variance in business and variance in statistics. From a business definition perspective variance is the difference between an observed value and an expected value. Within statistics, variance is a measure of variability around a mean. From a statistical perspective variance is used to determine statistical significance. See Figure 3.1 for the formulas for variance and standard deviation.

The nuances between variance and standard deviation from an interpretation standpoint are important to distinguish. Standard deviation is easier to interpret than variance. For example, a mean readmission rate of 12% with a standard deviation of 2% is interpreted using one standard deviation as a readmission rate between 10% and 14%. The calculation for variance would be 4 units squared, which is not in the same units as standard deviation. This minor nuance is easy

Sample Variance   **Sample Standard Deviation**

$$s^2 = \frac{\sum(x - \bar{x})^2}{n - 1} \qquad s = \sqrt{\frac{\sum(x - \bar{x})^2}{n - 1}}$$

Figure 3.1 Variance and standard deviation formulas.

to understand when the standard deviation is large but could easily be confused with a small standard deviation. Consider an example of a patient population with a mean age of 63.8 years and standard deviation of 14.3 years, which results in a variance of 204.5. The challenge is when the standard deviation is small. For example, a 7-point Likert-type scale with an average of 4.3 and standard deviation of 0.7 results in a variance of 0.49.

The interquartile range is the final measure of dispersion where a dataset is divided into quartiles split by the 25th, 50th, and 75th percentiles. The calculation of the interquartile range is the difference between the 75th and 25th quartiles. The larger the difference, the more variability within the data. The interquartile range is the building block of the box-and-whiskers plot, which displays the 25th, 50th (or median), and 75th percentiles along with the range of values or whiskers that displays the spread of data. Any value beyond the range or whiskers is considered an outlier.

Parametric/Non-parametric Statistics

The next step beyond the individual statistical concepts is the question of determining statistical significance. From a 50,000-foot perspective, statistics are initially categorized as quantitative (i.e., analyze numbers) or qualitative (i.e., analyze words). The primary focus is on quantitative statistics, but those interested in qualitative analyses are encouraged to consult a qualitative statistics textbook. Statistical concepts build on each other where previously discussed concepts (i.e., measures of central tendency/variability) are utilized in the formulas.

The next phase of demystifying statistics begins with breaking down quantitative statistical analyses into two categories: **parametric** and **non-parametric** statistics. The differentiation between parametric and non–parametric statistics is normally distributed data or a bell–shaped curve. Parametric statistics relies on normally distributed data and non-parametric statistics does not have this restriction. Regardless of quantitative/qualitative or parametric/non-parametric statistics, the end result is conducting statistical analyses to determine the significance of results to tell a story.

There are many statistical concepts or various buzz words gaining traction in healthcare to tell a story from numbers, such as machine learning, artificial intelligence, predictive analytics, prediction, modeling, predictive modeling, risk adjustment, risk adjustment model, etc. A technique that desires to predict an outcome is analyzed using regression models or referred to as **regression.** These predictions range from simple (i.e., predicting an outcome with one variable) to complex (i.e., predicting an outcome with multiple variables). Higher-level regression techniques, such as structural equation modeling or hierarchical linear modeling, examine even more complex relationships.

Regression

Regression is a statistical technique to predict a future outcome using the formula for a line ($y = mx + b$ or $y = ax + b$). Choosing a regression technique depends on the scale of measurement of the **criterion variable** or the outcome being predicted; for example, using nominal data where 1 is for an expired patient and 0 for an alive patient or 1 for a patient who keeps his/her scheduled appointment and 0 for a patient who does not keep his/her scheduled appointment. This type of a variable is a **dichotomous variable** or a nominal scale of measurement. Generally, a 1 indicates the presence of an event and a 0 indicates the absence of an event. The alternative to a dichotomous variable is a ratio or interval scale; these are **continuous variables.** Within regression, there are two outcomes: predicting dichotomous outcomes using **logistic regression** (i.e., predicting if a patient will expire or not) or continuous outcomes using **linear regression** (i.e., predicting a patient's length of stay). Remember, the scale of measurement of the outcome variable must be determined prior to choosing the regression type.

Logistic Regression

Logistic regression predicts categorical/dichotomous outcomes or nominal scales of measurement. The purpose is to determine what factors predict a specific event or outcome. For example, Parikh, George, Liyanage-Don, Hohler, Denis, and Weinberg (2017) utilized a logistic regression for a retrospective study involving stroke readmissions to determine interventions that may reduce readmissions. The purpose of the logistic regression is used to predict whether or not a patient will be readmitted based on demographic or clinical variables (i.e., age, comorbidities, insurances, distance, etc.) to determine if specific interventions may reduce the chances of being readmitted. Logistic regression results in a model or formula where a patient's characteristics can be put into the model to determine the probability of being readmitted.

Another application to logistic regression modeling is to generate an expected readmission rate that is used to calculate a risk-adjusted index to compare outcomes across hospitals. This risk-adjusted model alleviates criticism about readmission rates being higher at one hospital due to patients being sicker through controlling variables that may impact the outcome of interest. A caveat to this is that the logistic regression model is often based on administrative claims data, so information not documented in the patient's record by a coder cannot be included in a model. For example, there could be factors (i.e., eats meals high in sodium, no social support, not compliant with medications, body mass index, etc.) that are not documented, or they may be documented, but not coded. This would mean that some critical predictive readmission variables may not end up in administrative claims data. Developing risk-adjusted models is complex and complicated. What variables go into the regression model? Are there variables not captured that could explain the relationship?

A third application of logistic regression is a **k-means clustering model** in the statistical analysis of the Centers for Medicare/Medicaid Services (CMS) Star Rating. The methodology mathematically assigns a ranking, or in this case, a star rating, to combine multiple metrics assessed on different scales of measurement. For instance, readmission rate (percentages), average length of stay (days), infection rates (indices), and patient satisfaction scores (percentile ranks) are all measured using different scales. To statistically combine them for comparative purposes, all measures are standardized using a statistical procedure known as z-scoring. Once all z-scores are calculated, they can be combined. The CMS Star Rating (discussed further in Chapter 8) system used k-means clustering to create one overall star.

Linear Regression

Linear regression is like logistic regression because they both utilize statistical models to predict outcomes. The only difference is linear regression predicts a continuous outcome or a variable on an interval or ratio scale. There is no defined limit for the number of variables utilized to predict an outcome. However, from a psychological perspective, think about parsimony or simpler is better. The goal is to determine the least amount of variables that explain the majority of the outcome variable. For example, linear regression in healthcare is used to predict a patient's length of stay given a variety of clinical and demographic variables. Knowing that length of stay is a contributor to hospital cost makes it an important variable to study. Being able to understand the contributing factors for an increased length of stay creates the plausibility of aiming interventions towards reducing a patient's length of stay. Classen, Pestotnik, Evans, Lloyd, and Burke (1997) utilized linear regression to demonstrate that excess length of stay was due to adverse drug events. Similar to logistic regression, a linear regression results in a model where you can estimate a patient's length of stay based on the variables within the model.

Bridging the Gap between Statistical Methods and Healthcare

After reviewing predicting outcomes using logistic and linear regression, the next section introduces process and outcome variables within healthcare. Statistics in healthcare are everywhere; whether internal or external to the organization. Think about the publicly available CMS Star Ratings (Chapter 8) analyzing and weighting 60+ metrics to compare performance and rank hospitals. These metrics are unique to the star rating, but variations of those metrics impact other aspects of the organization and may appear in other initiatives that impact performance and financial outcomes. For example, the CMS Star Rating mortality domain has risk-adjusted mortality rates using the Medicare population, but hospitals treat all patients. Focusing on only the risk-adjusted metrics using the Medicare population only provides one side of the story. The Medicare population mortality rates from the regression model are then generalized (external validity) to the entire patient population. To complicate matters, CMS is one risk-adjusted methodology. Other organizations providing risk-adjusted data may use a different model than CMS. As mentioned in Chapter 1, hospitals have a responsibility for monitoring variations of the same metrics defined differently, so before interpreting, know your numbers and DEFINE your metrics. The methodology behind the data is important in understanding how to develop interventions to drive change.

You may encounter some metrics defined by the word rate, index, or ratio. Thinking methodologically about how these metrics are defined provides insight into how to interpret them. No specific rules exist on how those words are defined as it's up to the organization that created them to provide the definition. This could create issues as some organizations may use those three words interchangeably when they are calculated differently. Focusing on the methodology for defining each concept and knowing the data source is key to knowing the calculation for a rate, index, or ratio. When in doubt, DEFINE the metric. Let's start with some common definitions for rate, index, and ratio. Typically, a rate is multiplied by 100, an index is multiplied by 1,000 for easier interpretation with a large denominator, and a ratio is an observed rate divided by an expected rate. This serves as a general rule of thumb, because different data sources utilize the same word to mean something different.

Rates

Prior to analyzing any metric, think methodologically about the approach used to calculate that metric. One tool is to DEFINE a metric to understand the calculation or the "F" for factor and the "E" to evaluate the collected information for clarity. A **rate** is defined as a numerator divided by a denominator multiplied by 100. The interpretation of a rate is a metric per 100 discharges or a percentage. Some examples are a mortality rate, readmission rate, or surgical site infection rate. A value of 13 for readmissions is interpreted as 13 per 100 patient discharges or that 13% of patients are readmitted. This rate definition is incorrect for other data sources. For example, the CMS Star Rating includes a mortality rate, but the definition is a risk-adjusted rate using a regression model. The only way to know this is through a review of the methodology using the DEFINE tool. Regardless of the definition of a rate, the story originates from trending rates over time to infer trends or ask questions to understand what is happening.

Index

An **index** has multiple meanings depending on the data source, but analyzing the words preceding "index" provides a clue as to how it is calculated. An index is created when the denominator is large, so the calculation is a numerator divided by a denominator multiplied by 1,000. An example of an index is using infection statistics (i.e., intensive care unit (ICU) catheter-associated infection index or a non-ICU central line bacteremia index) from the National Healthcare Safety

Network (NHSN). The numerator is the number of infections and the denominator is patient care days, with the result multiplied by 1,000. An example interpretation would be 1.3 infections per 1,000 patient care days.

Using the index definition of multiplying the result by 1,000 leads to the wrong conclusion in two situations. The first is a *Clostridium difficile* (c diff or CDI) index within NHSN. The c diff index is calculated as the number of infections divided by patient care days multiplied by 10,000. The second is a risk-adjusted index where the numerator is an observed rate and denominator is an expected rate. A risk-adjusted mortality index means the numerator or observed rate is the total number of deaths divided by total number of discharges. The denominator or expected rate is risk-adjusted, utilizing logistic regression to control for variables impacting mortality, where an expected number of deaths is divided by total discharges. Dividing the observed rate by the expected rate results in a ratio of two percentages or a risk-adjusted index. A numerator or observed rate (i.e., 2.3%) that is the same as the denominator or expected rate (i.e., 2.3%) results in an index of 1.0. The interpretation of an index above 1.0 indicates performance is worse than expected or more patients died than were expected. An index below 1.0 indicates performance is better than expected or fewer patients died than were expected.

Ratio

The third statistical concept is a **ratio**. From a mathematical perspective, a ratio is a comparison between two non-zero values. These values are divided by each other to form a decimal, fraction, or percentage, with many definitions for ratios depending on the analyzed statistic. Similar to indices, pay attention to what precedes the word "ratio." Ratios are statistical in nature, such as an odds ratio, or specific to a metric, such as an NHSN standardized infection ratio (SIR). The statistical component of odds ratio is discussed later. The NHSN SIR metric is defined as a risk-adjusted ratio where the numerator is an observed number of infections and the denominator is an expected number of infections. Recall, this definition is the same as a risk-adjusted index, but NHSN uses the term ratio when referring to a risk-adjusted metric. This is why it's important to know the data source of your numbers and DEFINE the metric.

Rate, Index, and Ratio Trended Over Time

Leverage the power of statistics by incorporating multiple metrics to tell the whole story. Regardless of the metric analyzed, the end result of using statistics to tell a story is the same. One of the best predictors of future performance is past behavior (Wernimont & Campbell, 1968). Trending any of these statistics over time not only provides valuable insight into performance but can also provide additional questions. Trending data is done with any variation of time, such as annually, quarterly, monthly, weekly, daily, hourly, etc. to explore relationships and draw conclusions. Visually, **run charts** and **control charts** are two techniques for analyzing trends.

Run Charts

Run charts are used to monitor if trends are increasing or decreasing over time where the average rate/ratio/index is plotted along with the overall mean or median line. There are no restrictions to the minimum data points required for creating run charts. The decision for a mean or median line is based on the structure of the data. Datasets with outliers or extreme values may benefit from using the median. Datasets without outliers may benefit from using a mean. Run charts can be created in Microsoft Excel or any other report development software or statistical program. Keep in mind there are limitations to interpreting run charts. The only conclusion drawn is whether or not there is an increase or decrease over time following four rules:

1. Six or more consecutive points above or below the mean/median line
2. Run of 5 or more consecutive points ascending or descending
3. The amount of times the data crosses the mean/median line. Too many or too few can indicate a trend
4. An outlier that stands out from the rest. If standard deviation can be calculated on the dataset, then an outlier can be considered beyond the third standard deviation.

For example, Figure 3.2 provides a monthly rate for a metric. When analyzing this run chart, keep the rules in mind. The first rule is a trend of 6 or more consecutive data points above or below the mean/median. In this example, there are 7 points above the mean in the beginning of the run chart and 6 below the mean towards the end of the run chart. This indicates a potential change in process worth exploring to find out why. Rule 2 refers to an ascending or descending trend of 5 or more data points. The first 5 months of data are ascending, which indicates a change. It may be tempting to think the downward trend towards the end of the chart meets this rule, but there are points where the trend increases and decreases. While the general trend is decreasing, this would not violate a rule, but is worth further exploration. The third rule is how many times the data crosses the mean/median line. In this example, the data crosses the mean/median line 13 times out of 36 data points, which equates to 36.1% of data points. The question is, how many is too many? Not all rules are meant to be statistical. Remember to consider clinical significance as well and compare other metrics to determine how often data points cross the median/mean line in a similar timeframe. Do other metrics have the same percentage of data points crossing the line? With the fourth rule of outliers, this metric has a mean/median around 12. The highest value is around 17 and the lowest is around 8. This is where both clinical and statistical significance are important. A value of 17 or 8 could be above the third standard deviation, but in this example the standard deviation is unknown. Compare the high and low values of other metrics to gain an understanding of the variability and whether or not this is normal variation. The final point to consider is that any metric violating a clinical or statistical rule may or may not be negative. For

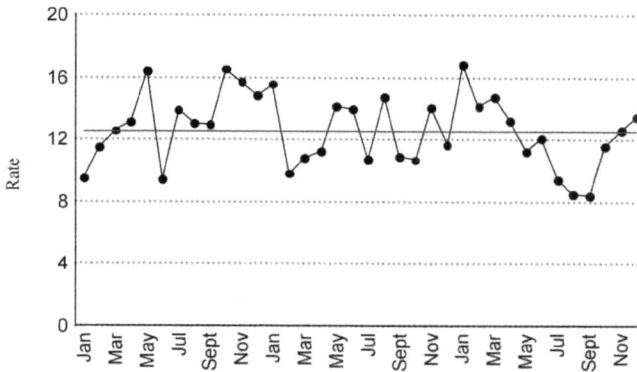

Figure 3.2 Run chart.

example, an outlier above the mean/median for patient experience means higher perceptions, which is positive.

Control Charts

Control charts build on the concept of run charts by adding the second and third standard deviation to the graph for additional insight and interpretation. One requirement for creating control charts is a minimum of 18 data points. There are three decisions to make when constructing a control chart: (1) use a median or mean line; (2) calculate fixed or floating standard deviations; and (3) select the type of control chart. The decision for a median or mean is based on the data being normally distributed. With skewed data or outliers the median or geometric mean may be a better representation of the data compared to the arithmetic mean. The second decision is choosing between setting floating limits where the standard deviation fluctuates over the timeframe or setting fixed limits where the standard deviation for the entire timeframe is calculated and plotted. Both have advantages and disadvantages. Calculating floating limits results in leveraging statistical knowledge to generate insight into your data. For example, think methodologically about the formula. The standard deviation denominator is sample size. A larger sample size equals a smaller standard deviation and a smaller sample size equals a larger standard deviation. Calculating a standard deviation on the entire timeframe, which likely equates to a large *n* size, may result in the standard deviation being closer to the mean or median. This could highlight more special cause violations due to the small standard deviation. Floating limits with standard deviation calculated monthly allows for examining the increase or decrease in monthly volume/sample size. This is an additional piece of information to leverage when methodologically approaching the analysis of a metric.

The purpose of two standard deviations on a control chart aligns with statistical probability, known as the normal curve or bell-shaped curve. Based on this concept two standard deviations capture about 95% of the variability and three standard deviations capture about 99% of the variability. Analyzing control chart variability is called common cause and special cause variation. Common cause variation is normal variation and accepted as typical fluctuation over time. Most healthcare professionals may not become alarmed with common cause variation. On the other hand, special cause variation requires additional exploration, knowing that 95% and 99% of all variation should be captured within 2 or 3 standard deviations. Statistically, special cause variation falls outside the statistical probability of occurrence. There may be more special cause rule violations, but here are eight rules of them:

1. A point outside the third standard deviation
2. Nine points in a row above or below the mean/median
3. Six consecutive points ascending or descending
4. Fourteen consecutive alternative points above or below the mean/median
5. Two out of 3 points beyond the second standard deviation
6. Four out of 5 points beyond the first standard deviation
7. Fifteen consecutive points above or below the first standard deviation
8. Eight consecutive points above or below the first standard deviation

Figure 3.3 provides examples of control charts with both fixed and floating limits. Using standard deviations as fixed limits may demonstrate special cause variation that doesn't exist within floating limits. Consider the few data points in the fixed limits that are beyond the third standard deviation, but do not appear beyond the third standard deviation of the floating limits. The interpretation of either the fixed or floating limits control charts is based on following the above eight rules. Adding standard deviation creates an additional interpretation of differentiating special cause variation from common cause variation. Common cause variation is considered normal fluctuations within the data that is due to error in measurement or minor changes in behavior over time. Special cause variation indicates that the fluctuations in the data are statistically different and would warrant an investigation into why. Keep in mind that not all special cause variation is negative. Having a compliance rate above the third standard deviation

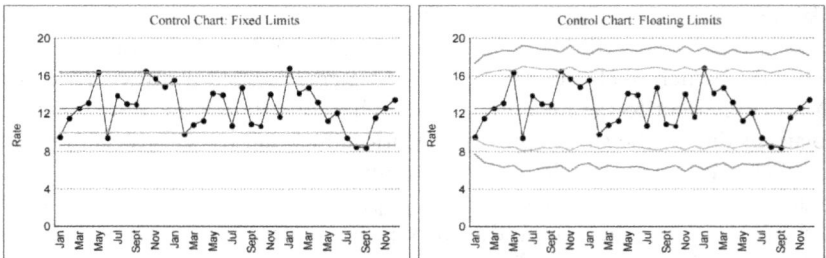

Figure 3.3 Control charts with fixed and floating limits.

is positive, but a mortality rate above the third standard deviation is a cause for concern.

The third question of choosing the type of control chart depends on the data. Control charts are based on chance or probability and not every event has the same probability of occurrence. How much data is collected and the scale of measurement of the data being collected impact the type of control chart that is used. Regardless of the nuances to the types of control charts, they all contain similar features of a mean/median and upper and lower control limits (i.e., standard deviations or standard errors). The calculations and interpretations may vary slightly, but the main purpose of common cause or special cause variation is a common characteristic of what makes a control chart. Readers interested in different types of control charts are advised to read Provost and Murray's (2011) *The Health Care Data Guide: Learning from Data for Improvement.*

Confidence Intervals

Another important and effective statistic is **confidence intervals**. These are calculated using a sample of data to estimate another sample or generalize to the population. The interpretation is to state, with confidence, that data collected from another sample would be within the calculated confidence interval. A word of caution when analyzing data is to know if you have the entire population or a sample. There is no need to calculate a confidence interval when analyzing the entire population, because the calculated metric is the population.

When calculating a confidence interval, it is advised to have a sample size above 30. The most common confidence intervals are 90%, 95%, and 99%, where 95% is used most frequently. The range of values within a confidence interval gets wider as the level of confidence increases from 90% to 99%. Important points to consider with confidence intervals are as follows:

1. Confidence intervals are used when a sample of data is collected with the desire to estimate a range within population.
2. Confidence intervals are used to determine statistical significance two ways: compared to external benchmarks (i.e., confidence interval must be completely above or below a benchmark to be significant) and the inclusion of a specific value (i.e., confidence interval includes 0, then it's not significant, or a confidence interval calculated on a risk-adjusted value that has 1.0 included is not significant).

Percentiles/Percentile Ranks

Percentiles and **percentile ranks** are useful to quantifiably compare relationships with the purpose of ranking outcomes within a larger dataset. For example, it doesn't matter whether you say a score of 89.5 on patient experience (Chapter 5) falls in the 45th percentile or an 89.5 score is in the 45th percentile rank, the percentile rank adds context to say this score is better than 45% of the hospitals in the national database. Percentile ranks provide benchmark information for organizations to assist in setting priorities and goals to strive towards the never-ending moving target. The one caveat is knowledge is powerful when leveraged appropriately. Knowing an organization's score falls in the 13th percentile doesn't provide enough information on how to improve. Thus, focusing improvement efforts on one metric only tells one piece of a larger puzzle. Leveraging the observed score used for the calculation of the percentile rank provides further insight into developing behavioral interventions to improve.

Odds Ratio

Odds ratios is the final statistical concept. The interpretation of an odds ratio depends on the statistical concept being analyzed. Odds ratios are found in two applications: (1) logistic regression; and (2) associations between variables. An odds ratio in logistic regression is interpreted as a measure of probability by asking: "what are the odds or probability a specific event occurs given a change in the predictor (independent) variable?" Remember, probability is the chance of an event happening that ranges between 0 and 1, where 0 is 0% chance of an event happening and 1 is 100% chance of an event happening. The odds ratio in logistic regression is a measure of the probability of success divided by the probability of failure. The interpretation for odds ratio in logistic regression is when a value is above 1 there is a greater chance of the outcome of interest occurring and a value less than 1 means there is less of a chance for the outcome of interest to occur.

The second application is a measure of association between two events. These two events could be a 2×2, which consists of two different variables comprised of two different groups. The Institute for Healthcare Improvement (IHI) developed a 2×2 methodology to review patients who were admitted/not admitted to an ICU and did/did not have comfort care. The odds ratio is a measure of association between these events that is tested statistically using a chi-square statistic.

Conclusion

Statistics are around us all the time and may often be overlooked, because decisions we make may not involve a formula. We may simply say, "If I leave my house by 7am, then I will be at work by 8am." This mental calculation is leveraging probability to determine the success of arriving at work on time without utilizing a formula to calculate the specific probability. Don't worry if you don't remember/understand each statistical concept because this chapter was meant to provide a summary of common statistics within healthcare. Each subsequent chapter focuses on a specific healthcare topic to integrate research methodology and statistics to provide insight for setting goals and managing change through behavioral interventions. Although methodologies between analytics and research vary, understanding the methodology behind the statistics transcends all healthcare topics by breaking complex processes into manageable pieces.

Our goal is to teach an applied methodological approach to statistical evaluation to enhance your confidence in storytelling with statistics. At the conclusion of this book, you will have the knowledge/skill to: know your numbers, ask the right questions to develop behavioral interventions, and set goals using sound methodology to drive and monitor change. Learning these skills will help hit those moving targets on your way to number 1. Disclaimer: following all advice in this book will not guarantee you will reach number 1, because there's only one person/place that occupies the top spot.

Discussion Questions

- Do you believe statistics provide answers or more questions?
- Given the definitions of type I and type II error, would you rather be told that something works when it doesn't or that something doesn't work when it does?
- Do you believe in collecting as much data as possible in order to make the best statistical decision?
- Have you ever made an improvement decision that didn't work as expected and tried to understand why?
- We may operate under the assumption that more is always better: collect more data over a longer period of time to have the most amount of data to make the best decision. Sometimes the best intentions may not work. What are your thoughts on collecting as much data as possible vs. using a power analysis to determine how many you need for significance?
- Sometimes individuals analyzing data and clinicians may clash on what is considered significant. In your experience, have you encountered a situation where something was statistically significant and not clinically significant or vice versa. What did you do?
- What are the benefits of using a run chart or control chart?
- How would you create a story around special cause variations in Figure 3.3?

4 Mortality and Readmission

"How you do something is equally as important as how well you do something."

Introduction

There are many philosophies about initiating change. Have you ever thought about or said any of the following? If something is not documented, then it's not done. If it's not measured, then there is no way to improve. You can't manage something if it's not measured. Not measuring something means it is not possible to change it. Whatever statement rings true, the general theme is that driving change requires measurement. This framework is the concept of input → process → outcome. We think of something (input), we do something (process), then something happens (outcome). This simplistic view is more complex in practice, because no single input impacts a single process to result in only one outcome. The complex world we live in more likely results in intertwined inputs and processes with complex outcomes.

Taking a step back and focusing on a methodological approach results in measuring healthcare variables using two broad categories: **process metrics** and **outcome metrics**. From a statistical perspective, understanding both process and outcomes creates a better picture of what is happening within an organization. Regardless of the type of metric analyzed, both are used to trend, monitor, and evaluate various processes/outcomes of interest. A process metric is "how you do something" and the outcome metric is "how well you did something." In other words, a process metric involves the steps leading up to an event and an outcome metric is the result of what happened after the process was completed. Both process and outcome metrics are important to understand because improving an outcome requires an understanding of the process utilized for that outcome.

Think of process metrics as the method used to arrive at an outcome. Process metrics capture the operational performance of an organization in an effort to improve efficiency and effectiveness through a series of measuring the steps involved. An example of a process metric is calculating the average time it takes to administer antibiotics to determine the impact on mortality. In this example, antibiotic administration is a process, because the end result or outcome is mortality. The antibiotic administration is one of many steps or processes that have an impact on an outcome.

Outcome metrics are utilized to understand organizational accountability and demonstrate how well or poorly organizations do with respect to performance on some metric. An outcome metric is the end result of a process metric or what happens as a result of a particular event. An example of an outcome metric is a mortality or readmission rate. These are considered outcome metrics as this is the end result of a series of processes or steps taken. Stepping outside healthcare, think of all the steps that go into starting a vehicle. The main outcome of interest is whether or not the vehicle starts. Every step that occurs before the vehicle starts consists of a measurable process metric to analyze when the outcome (i.e., vehicle starts) fails.

A factor that adds complexity to the process of care delivery is a patient's desire to be involved in the decision-making process, which is referred to as shared decision making, patient-, person-, or family-centered care. Regardless of the semantics, the outcome is to incorporate patients into the care delivery process. Mixed results exist about the utility of this approach; Waterworth and Luker (1990) concluded that patients may comply with doing what is right or what the clinician deems appropriate. Promoting individualized care for patients is not the same as having patients actively involved in the decision-making process. Within the intensive care unit (ICU) less than half of patients included expressed a desire to participate in the decision-making process and only 15% actually participated (Azoulay, Pochard, Chevret, Adrie, Annane, Bleichner, … & Goldgran-Toledano, 2004). The needs of a patient come first, so the concept of patient-centered care isn't new (Berwick, 2009). A plausible rationale for why shared decision making rarely happens is because it's hard to implement and not taught (Godolphin, 2009).

Healthcare should not be viewed as a one-way street. Despite these findings, patients are encouraged to become active participants in the delivery of their care (Epstein & Street, 2011; Reynolds, 2009) to promote patient-centered care or shared decision making (Barry & Edgman-Levitan, 2012). The care being delivered directly impacts the patient and evidence-based care promotes the use of shared decision making for patient safety, improved compliance, and reducing adverse events (Godolphin, 2009). The Institute for Healthcare Improvement (IHI) provides resources to organizations seeking to be patient-centered (Frampton, Guastello, Brady, Hale, Horowitz, Bennett Smith, & Stone, 2008) and emphasizes the importance of providing person- and family-centered care to honor the requests of individual patients.

With that said, outcome metrics are forward-facing metrics seen by the public and other organizations that reflect how a hospital is performing. It's possible that, from a patient's perspective, the most important metric is the overall outcome or end result, but patient involvement in the care delivery process is vital and may impact other unintended outcomes (i.e., satisfaction with communication). The steps or processes leading up to the event are critical to ensure a positive outcome, but the main focus may be on the outcome. The point is there are many processes that must occur prior to the outcome and any process breakdown may impact the end result. Outcome metrics may be easier to measure and explain to others, which makes them easy targets for a financial or performance impact. With the evolution of healthcare from a fee-for-service (FFS) to being paid for performance, these outcome metrics become critical as governmental and other organizations focus less on process and more on outcome to drive accountability along the entire continuum of care.

The one caveat to improve an outcome metric is to understand the process for two reasons: (1) outcome metrics drive financial reimbursement; and (2) process metrics drive quality of care. As a result, focusing on both reasons to improve is necessary. Additionally, we never know where the future of healthcare may go, but having metrics (i.e., process and/or outcome) to evaluate performance is inevitable. Before determining methods to monitor, trend, and evaluate metrics, understand the impact that process and outcome metrics have on organizations. Many organizations/initiatives utilize both process and outcome metrics to drive improvement and efficiency, including: Centers for Medicare/Medicaid Services (CMS), Department of Health (DOH), Joint Commission, Agency for Healthcare Research and Quality (AHRQ), IHI, Press Ganey, Value-Based Purchasing (VBP), Bundled Payments, Partnership for Patients, Pay for Performance (P4P), Star Rating, etc. The list could continue, but the message is clear. Improving outcomes and processes drives accountability from both a quality/financial perspective and impacts organizational performance. Remember the key to knowing your numbers is to DEFINE the metrics being analyzed to better understand what is being measured.

An unlimited amount of process and outcome metrics exists within healthcare, so it is not feasible to measure, analyze, and change everything. From a methodological perspective, the DEFINE tool enhances an understanding of the operationalization of a metric (i.e., enhances construct validity). Methodology combined with statistics eliminates subjectivity and objectively analyzes data to focus on the FACTS.

- F: Formulas – identify the formulas for the calculation of the statistics presented.
- A: Analyze patterns/trends – examine variability within the data.
- C: Consider guidelines/rules – determine any guidelines/rules for interpretation.
- T: Think – take time to think about what the data is objectively showing.
- S: Statistics – determine the statistics being used to test your creativity.

Trending metrics over time is an effective way to understand patterns and be proactive with implementing future change. Two previously discussed graphical tools for trending, monitoring, and evaluating data that can be used for mortality and readmission rates are **run charts** or **control charts**. Keep in mind that other graphical ways to present data effectively exist, such as a **bar graph**, a **pie chart**, a **Pareto chart**, or a **scatter plot**. The choice is up to you as to how to creatively display data to maximize effectiveness and tell the story.

Run/Control Chart Contradiction

The purpose of graphic displays is to provide a backdrop for storytelling, but there are a couple of challenges with this. With respect to process and outcome metrics, process metrics use control charts to identify variation within an existing process. The argument over whether or not a control chart is useful for outcome metrics (i.e., readmissions or mortalities) is debatable. The counterargument to using control charts for monitoring outcome metrics is wondering if a better graphical alternative exists. Regardless of your view, control charts are created with continuous (i.e., antibiotic administration time) or discrete (i.e., readmitted or not) data. Discrete readmission data is converted to rates (0–100%) for purposes of telling a story and to calculate a mean and standard deviation. The important point to consider is that many process metrics can impact one outcome metric, so a further analysis is warranted for readmission rates to determine how to improve performance based on special cause variation highlighted in the control chart.

The other challenge is the number of data points recommended for analyzing trends. There is no limit to the amount of data points displayed using a run chart, whereas a minimum of 18 points is recommended for creating control charts. Keep in mind that having more than 18 points is not a guarantee for utilizing a control chart. Control charts require calculating standard deviation. The formula for calculating standard deviation requires an average value, observed value, and a total sample size. To calculate these, you need raw data for every individual in a dataset. Without the raw individual level data, standard deviation may not be calculated. Leverage the DEFINE tool to compare and contrast the risk-adjusted readmission index to the readmission rate to better understand the calculations behind these metrics (Table 4.1).

Table 4.1 DEFINE tool comparison

Tool	Readmission rate	Risk-adjusted readmission index
D – Denominator	All patients eligible for being readmitted to your organization	Expected readmission rate – calculated by the number of expected readmissions divided by all patients eligible and multiplied by 100
E – Exclusion criteria	Any patient not eligible for readmission. This could exclude patients that expired, or certain clinical decisions for exclusion (i.e., planned admissions). Centers for Medicare/Medicaid Services (CMS) has a list of planned readmissions	
F – Factor	Since this is a readmission rate, the calculation is multiplied by 100	No multiplication. It is a ratio of the observed rate divided by the expected rate
I – Inclusion criteria	There was no specific reference to a patient population like heart failure or pneumonia, so any patient diagnosis would be included	
N – Numerator	Any patient readmitted to the hospital for any reason within 30 days of being discharged	Observed readmission rate – calculated by the total number of readmissions divided by all patients eligible and multiplied by 100
E – Evaluate	The readmission rate is a percentage of all patients readmitted to the hospital within 30 days for any reason, with the exception of patients who expired on the current admission or any planned readmission, as applicable	The risk-adjusted readmission index is a ratio of an observed rate divided by an expected rate to compare performance

Before analyzing why this can or cannot be done, recall the risk-adjusted readmission index is a ratio of an observed readmission rate to an expected readmission rate. The expected readmission rate is calculated by a logistic regression model that takes into consideration variables that influence the outcome variable. Risk adjustment relies on administrative billing data to adjust for variables impacting the outcome. The overall index allows for comparisons across different hospitals (i.e., tertiary vs. community hospitals) or patient characteristics (i.e., older vs. younger patients). The general interpretation is an index above 1.0 indicates performance is worse than expected and an index below 1.0 indicates performance is better than expected. Why?

For argument's sake, an observed readmission rate is 12% and an expected readmission rate is 18%. The result of dividing 12% by 18% is 0.67, which is the index. In other words, the interpretation is 18% of patients were expected to be readmitted, but 12% were readmitted, which is better than was expected. Likewise, if an observed readmission rate was 22% and an expected readmission rate was still 18%, then the index would be 1.22. This means more patients were readmitted than were expected to be.

How does this relate to what is needed for calculating a standard deviation and creating a control chart? A control chart relies on the calculation of the second and third standard deviation for interpreting special or common cause variation. Access to the raw data becomes critical. With the readmission rate, the numerator and denominator are individual people, which is the lowest unit of analysis and provides the ability to calculate standard deviation. With the risk-adjusted readmission index, the numerator is an observed rate calculated by the total number of patients readmitted divided by the total number of patients eligible for readmission. The denominator is an expected rate calculated by the total number of patients expected to be readmitted divided by the total number of patients eligible for readmission. Since the numerator and denominator are calculated rates, it is not possible to determine what the total sample size is. Therefore, standard deviation cannot be calculated. The following two paragraphs present two different scenarios critically thinking about the data and formulas.

In this example we use 2 months of data to illustrate the point as to why a risk-adjusted index alone cannot be used to calculate standard deviation. To add context, the readmission rate is compared with the risk-adjusted readmission index (Table 4.2). In the readmission rate, the numerator for January is 25 and February is 21, which combined sums to 46. The denominator for January

Table 4.2 Readmission rate and risk-adjusted readmission index example

Time	Readmission rate			Risk-adjusted readmission index		
	Numerator	Denominator	Rate	Numerator	Denominator	Index
January	25	300	8.3%	12.2%	10%	1.22
February	21	150	14%	9%	11.8%	0.76
Total	46	450	10.2%	12.1%	10.7%	1.13

$$\overline{X} = \frac{\sum X}{N}$$

Figure 4.1 Mean or average formula.

is 300 and February is 150, which combined sums to 450. Therefore, the mean is 46/450 or 10.2%. Risk-adjusted data is calculated through a regression model by the company that created it. In the risk-adjusted index example, the numerator for January is 12.2% and denominator is 10%. When dividing these two values the resulting index is 1.22. For February, the numerator is 9% and the denominator is 11.8%. The result is an index of 0.76. In both months, the values for the numerators and denominators are already calculated rates. There is no way to sum up the numerators or denominators to calculate an average.

One additional piece of information was intentionally left out of the risk-adjusted readmission index example. When risk-adjusted information is often provided, the software will provide an overall sample size. For example, assume the provided sample size for the risk-adjusted readmission index for Month A is 500 with an observed rate of 12.2% and expected rate of 10%, resulting in a 1.22 index. Leveraging the mean formula from Figure 4.1 indicates that two of the three values are available for the risk-adjusted readmission index. The only value not provided is the numerator of the mean formula or the total number or people. Knowing that the observed rate for Month A is 12.2% and the *n* size is 500, multiplying 12.2% by 500 to solve for the number of readmits would give 61. Applying the logic to the expected rate for Month A of 10% and an *n* size of 500 results in 50 expected readmits. We can convert the observed (12.2%) and expected (10%) rates to observed ($n = 61$) and expected ($n = 50$) readmissions. Step back and focus on the provided 1.22 index. Mathematically, the end result (1.22) is the same when dividing 12.2% by 10% or 61 by 50. The advantage to having the raw numbers means that it's possible to use the raw numbers and calculate standard deviation. This calculation, with a little creativity, makes it possible to convert a risk-adjusted readmission index from a run chart into a control chart by being able to calculate standard deviation.

Methodologically Testing Your Creativity with Data

While the purpose of graphical displays is to answer questions, sometimes data generates more questions than answers. The only limit to interpreting data is your own objective creativity. As a reminder, not all special cause variation indicates poor performance and some common cause variation may be concerning. Does consistent performance lead to a top performer? At this point, step back and think methodologically about the potential analysis of a metric and setting a goal. Think about the formulas being introduced and test your creativity with the data to move beyond what is provided. When analyzing risk-adjusted readmission indices, the values typically provided are the observed rate (numerator), expected rate (denominator), index, and the total sample (*n*) size. Leveraging a formula and being creative can make what seems impossible possible.

Run Charts Methodology

Run charts are graphical representations of data used to monitor trends/patterns within data. Similar to the statistics discussed in Chapter 3, there are varying degrees of complexity and some statistics build on other statistics. The main components for a run chart are an *x*-axis variable, which is generally time broken down into hours, days, weeks, months, quarters, years, or any variation for trending time, and the *y*-axis variable, which is the trended process or outcome metric. The final component is plotting the overall mean/average or median.

Once you DEFINE your metric of interest, the process begins with plotting time (i.e., months) on the *x*-axis. The *y*-axis variable is a monthly readmission rate. We never want to jump to conclusions with making decisions, so take a step back and think about the methodological process of what goes into a readmission rate before analyzing trends. In this example, we DEFINE readmission as follows:

D: Denominator – all patients eligible for being readmitted to an organization.

E: Exclusion criteria – any patient not eligible. This could be excluding patients who died, or certain planned admissions (psychiatric, chemical dependency, or rehabilitation). CMS has a list of planned readmissions built in their readmission algorithm.

F: Factor – a readmission rate is calculated by multiplying the result by 100.

I: Inclusion criteria – there was no specific reference to a patient population like heart failure or pneumonia, so any patient diagnosis is included.

N: Numerator – any patient readmitted to the same hospital for any reason within 30 days of being discharged.

E: Evaluate – the readmission rate is a percentage of all patients readmitted to the same hospital within 30 days, for any reason, with the exception of patients who expired on the current admission or any planned readmission, as applicable.

Run Chart Results

After fully understanding the readmission metric from a methodological perspective, the next step is to examine the methodology of a run chart. The purpose of a run chart is to indicate whether or not a specific trend is increasing or decreasing (www.qualitydigest.com/inside/quality-insider-article/making-and-interpreting-run-charts.html). As mentioned in Chapter 3, there are four run chart rules to identify trends.

1. A **shift** of 6 or more consecutive points above or below the mean, where values that fall on the mean are skipped.

2. A **trend** of 5 or more consecutive points increasing or decreasing, where 2 or more successive points that are the same are ignored.
3. A **run** of 5 data points above or below the mean line, where an indicator of change would be 1 or many runs crossing the mean line.
4. An **astronomical point** that is extremely large or small, which is classified as an outlier.

The creation of a run chart can be accomplished using various tools, such as Microsoft Excel, Minitab, SPSS, SAS, Crystal Reports, Tableau, Qlikview, R, etc.

Figure 4.2 is an overall monthly readmission rate run chart. The fluctuating line indicates the monthly rate and the single straight line represents the overall mean/average over that particular time period. Prior to analyzing data, focus on the FACTS presented:

1. Formulas – average rate and rate calculated by summing the numerator and dividing by the sum of the denominator.
2. Analyze patterns and trends – overall trend is down with a slight increasing trend towards the end. Additionally, there is some variability with months increasing and decreasing.
3. Consider guidelines/rules – based on the four rules for interpretation, there is a shift/trend with more than 5 consecutive points below the mean and an astronomical point.
4. Think – don't jump to conclusions and focus on the entire graph. While it appears there is a decreasing trend from the beginning to the end, there may be some cause for concern with the rising trend towards the end (last 8 points).
5. Statistics – run charts display rates and means. Knowing that the average can be influenced by outliers is an important consideration to decide on a mean or median.

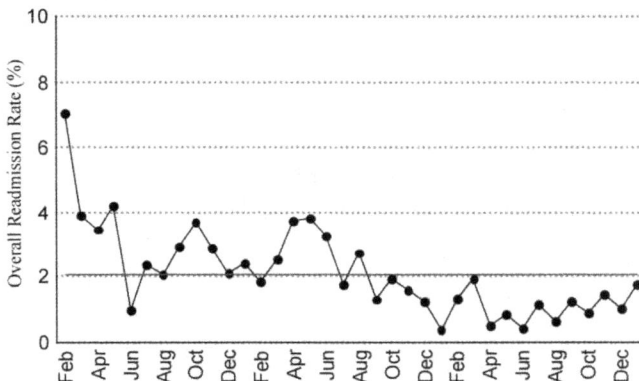

Figure 4.2 Run chart example.

After focusing on the FACTS, the next step is an objective story. The overall readmission rate is decreasing over time with some variability up and down throughout the timeframe. More importantly, there are two rules that identify important interpretation points from the analysis. They are the astronomical point in the beginning and the shift/trend of more than 5 consecutive points below the mean at the end. One potential consideration about the astronomical point of around 7% is that the mean is influenced by outliers. Knowing that the rate is comprised of the sum of the numerator divided by the sum of the denominator, this high rate could be influenced by outliers that may be different from the other months. It's worthwhile investigating this further. Were there fewer patients that month? Were there outside factors (i.e., severe weather) that were beyond your control? Were patients more critically complex? Secondly, even though there is a shift/trend with more than 5 consecutive points below the mean, towards the end of the graph the months alternate up and down with the overall trend appearing to move towards the mean. While it may be tempting to celebrate the accomplishment of having a monthly average below the overall mean, the upward trend could indicate a potential breakdown in process resulting in minor monthly increases. This may also be worthwhile investigating further as it is not a specific rule for interpretation, but with time could be problematic.

Control Chart Methodology

The other graphical representation is a control chart. Many different types of control charts exist based on the type of data (discrete or continuous). Interested readers could consult Provost and Murray's (2011) book titled *The Health Care Data Guide: Learning from Data for Improvement* for choosing the type of control chart you give your data. From a statistical perspective, there are different probabilities of events occurring that comprise various probability distributions, which results in different calculations. The implication is that event probability for purposes of creating a control chart impacts how the control limits are created.

There are similarities between run and control charts, but enhancements are added to control charts that allow for a different interpretation. A control chart has two minor distinctions:

1. To effectively utilize a control chart a minimum of 18 data points is recommended.
2. Control limits or standard deviations are added to the trends where the second and third standard deviation are commonly plotted.

Before getting into the methodology of control charts, it's important to discuss the rationale behind why and how the standard deviations are used. Recall from Chapter 3 that standard deviation in statistics is a measure of dispersion around the mean. In other words, it's a measure of how much variability exists within the analyzed data. Another concept is the normal distribution/bell-shaped curve/

normal curve, whereby variability captured within 1 standard deviation is about 68%, within 2 standard deviations is 95%, and within 3 standard deviations is 99%. There is an added advantage of analyzing data utilizing this knowledge because, statistically, 95–99% of variability is captured within 2–3 standard deviations.

Recall from Chapter 3 that we discussed two options for plotting standard deviations in a control chart: (1) create fixed limits, where the standard deviation is calculated for the entire timeframe (Figure 4.3); or (2) calculate floating limits, where the standard deviation is calculated based on the time interval on the *x*-axis (Figure 4.4). Either option results in a story, but critical information is lost when using fixed vs. floating standard deviations.

There is an additional third option for calculating control limits when using statistical process control programs where fixed control limits are recalculated at

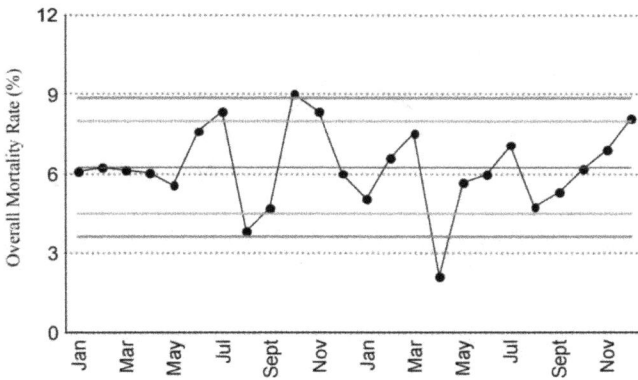

Figure 4.3 Control chart with fixed limits.

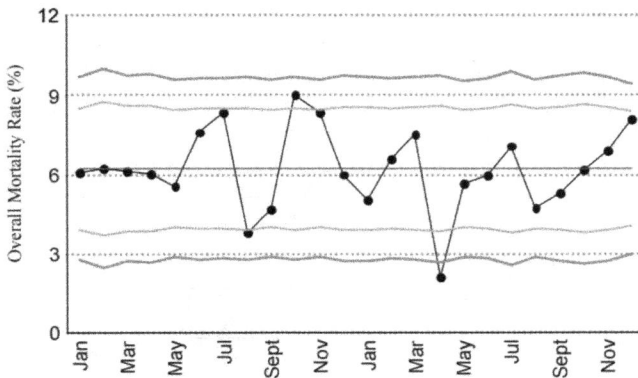

Figure 4.4 Control chart with floating limits.

the point where special cause variation occurs. For example, when an intervention is implemented to reduce mortality rates, an approach could be to use fixed limits before and after to monitor change. For example, Figure 4.5 monitors sepsis mortality over time with multiple interventions using fixed limits. The downside to fixed limits is that a larger sample size results in smaller standard deviations. The end result is a control limit close to the mean that may indicate special cause variation when it may not be true (remember type II error).

An alternative to the fixed limits is to create floating limits where the standard deviation is calculated based on each individual time period as opposed to performance over an entire interval. This results in the ability to examine fluctuations in monthly variability and a standard deviation less likely to be influenced by a large sample. For example, Figure 4.6 contains a control chart with floating limits

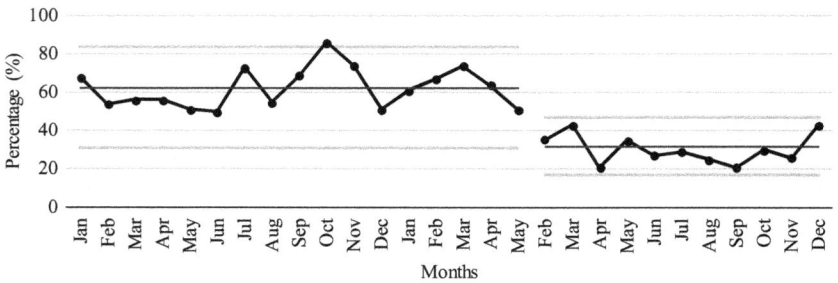

Figure 4.5 Sepsis mortality with re-calculated fixed limits.

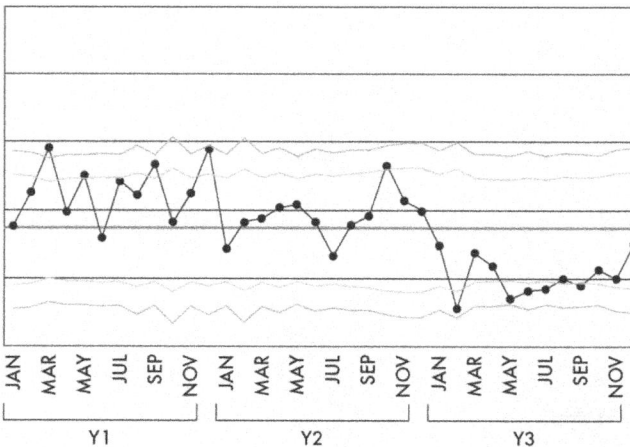

Figure 4.6 Sepsis mortality with floating limits.

for sepsis mortality. When reviewing the control chart using fixed limits, there are monthly data points that are identified as being special cause variation, but using floating limits results in no special cause. A plausible explanation (i.e., threat to validity) is due to calculating standard deviation for the entire time period instead of monthly.

In the end, the decision of whether to use Figure 4.5 or 4.6 is up to you. There are advantages and disadvantages to both. The most important point is knowing your audience and presenting the most effective story. Let's take a further look at how the standard deviation calculation varies using the monthly vs. entire timeframe. The standard deviation is calculated based on four different sample sizes (50, 100, 150, and 1,500) for the total timeframe. The numerator for the standard deviation formula will remain constant at 450. The standard deviation with a sample size of 50 is 3.0, for a sample size of 100 is 2.1, and 1.7 for a sample of 150. Comparing these standard deviations to a fixed limit with a larger sample size ($n = 1,500$) would result in a 0.5 standard deviation.

Given an average severe sepsis mortality rate of 23.0% means that a special cause variation beyond 3 SD would differ based on a sample size of 50, 100, 150, or 1,500 (Table 4.3). Using a sample size of 50, a special cause variation is a mortality rate above 32.0% (23.0% plus 9.0% for 3 SD), for a sample size of 100 is above 29.3% (23.0% plus 6.3% for 3 SD), for a sample size of 150 is 28.1% (23.0% plus 5.1% for 3 SD), and lastly a sample size of 1,500 would result in a mortality rate of 24.5% (23.0% plus 1.5 for 3 SD). Depending on sample size, what is considered special cause (i.e., beyond the third standard deviation) is 32%, 29.3%, 28.1%, or 24.5%. Given this hypothetical scenario, this simulation shows the how sample size influences standard deviation, which can impact special cause variation interpretation.

Knowing the relationship between sample size and its impact on standard deviation allows you to gain further insight on variation in volume over time. Extremely wide control limits or standard deviation may be indicative of a smaller volume whereas standard deviation close to the mean could be indicative of a larger volume. This knowledge could help you make the decision on graphing fixed or floating limits! Seeing fluctuations in limits may be a sign of inconsistency between monthly volume, which could prompt a question of how can we be consistent over time with fluctuation in monthly volume? This drives the question away from increasing or decreasing a rate and focuses more on the population within your metric. A fixed limit, on the other hand, does not allow for

Table 4.3 Standard deviation example with increasing sample sizes

Average	$\Sigma (x-x)2$	n	Standard deviation	3 SD
23.0	450	50	3.0	9.0
23.0	450	100	2.1	6.3
23.0	450	150	1.7	5.1
23.0	450	1,500	0.5	1,5

interpretation of variability of the volume between data points, which may be OK with the story you are telling.

When examining variability, the two types discussed in Chapter 3 were: (1) common cause variation; and (2) special cause variation. Common cause variation is normal fluctuations between data points that occur as a result of natural variations. Most common cause variation may not be a major concern, but this doesn't imply that common cause variation can be ignored and deemed normal variation. Since the second standard deviation captures approximately 95% of the variability and the third standard deviation captures approximately 99% of the variability, special cause variation rules were developed to further explore. The following are eight special cause variation rules:

1. Any point outside the control limits
2. 9 points in a row on the same side of the center line
3. 6 points in a row increasing or decreasing
4. 14 points in a row alternating up or down
5. 2 of 3 points beyond 2 SD from the mean
6. 4 of 5 points beyond 1 SD from the mean
7. 15 points in a row less than 1 SD from the mean
8. 8 points in a row beyond 1 SD from the mean.

Control Chart Results

For the results of a control chart, the analysis utilizes the monthly overall mortality rate using both fixed limits (Figure 4.3) and floating limits (Figure 4.4). The interpretation of a control chart with fixed limits vs. floating limits is similar, but minor variations occur based on special cause variation rules and fluctuation in monthly volume inferred from standard deviation.

When analyzing Figure 4.3 with fixed standard deviation limits, the first October point is beyond the third standard deviation, which violates rule 1 (any point beyond the third standard deviation). In reviewing the same point in the floating limits, there is no special cause variation for the first October point. Why? Remember, the denominator of standard deviation is n size or sample size. Knowing fixed limits use the sample size for the entire time period and floating limits use the sample size for each individual month, this is one cause of why fixed limits are closer to the mean than floating limits. Always remember to DEFINE the metric before focusing on the FACTS.

1. Formulas − standard deviation utilizes raw numbers and the n size or sample size, average monthly rate, and overall average calculated by summing the numerator divided by the sum of the denominator.
2. Analyze patterns/trends − fluctuation within standard deviation limits, trends appear to increase and decrease over time with an increasing trend towards the end.
3. Consider guidelines/rules − the second April point is beyond the third standard deviation and the last 5 points are increasing. Majority monthly data falls within common cause variation.

4. Think – knowing that the last 5 points are increasing, consider special cause variation; what other variables may influence mortality rates over time? What process metrics may help? Why was there a change in volume on a monthly basis? Is this a metric that impacts financial incentives or is included in publicly reported performance scores?
5. Statistics – control charts display rates, means, and standard deviation.

These FACTS provide critical information on where to focus future initiatives. The first point is examining fluctuations in standard deviation. What does it mean when there is monthly variation on volume? Why were there fewer/more patients during a given month? Yes, there is a lot of common cause variation, but does common cause variation lead to becoming a top performer? Can common cause variation turn into special cause if it's discounted as normal fluctuation? Is the hospital currently stuck with their current performance and is this a good thing? How can process metrics be developed to improve a seemingly stagnant trend? The second April point was below the lower third standard deviation, which violates special cause variation, and the volume of patients that month was consistent with previous months. What happened that month and why was the mortality rate low? The last 5 months are trending up, which may not violate special cause rules now. Why not be proactive instead of reactive and think about what you can do to avoid a future special cause violation while it's common cause?

Discussion

Developing a graphical representation (i.e., run and control charts) of data over time is effective to tell a story with data. Visually inspecting patterns/trends may be easier to interpret than looking at only numbers. In the beginning of this chapter, the focus was on process and outcome metrics and how they are utilized for monitoring, trending, and evaluating financial improvement or quality of care outcomes. The middle portion of the chapter focused on the methodology and results for run charts and control charts separately. The final portion of this chapter focuses on the bigger picture and tests your creativity through understanding the data by focusing on the FACTS.

When collecting information to diagnose a patient, do you focus on one symptom or a variety of symptoms, including other critical variables? Jumping to conclusions on a diagnosis may lead to no further critical thinking (i.e., does thinking stop when a diagnosis is made?). Diagnosing a patient with one symptom could lead to the incorrect diagnosis, so how can improvement decisions be made using only one metric (i.e., raw mortality rate)? The answer is, the raw mortality rate only tells one piece of the puzzle, which is how many people expired in that analysis. It doesn't tell you anything about process or comorbidities or risk of mortality or individual patient characteristics. However, daily decisions are made using one piece of information. In order to tell a story of what is happening and set a goal, leverage as many metrics as possible to tell a more complete story than only one metric can do. This could mean integrating outcome metrics, such as the observed rate and the risk-adjusted index or incorporating process metrics that may impact an outcome.

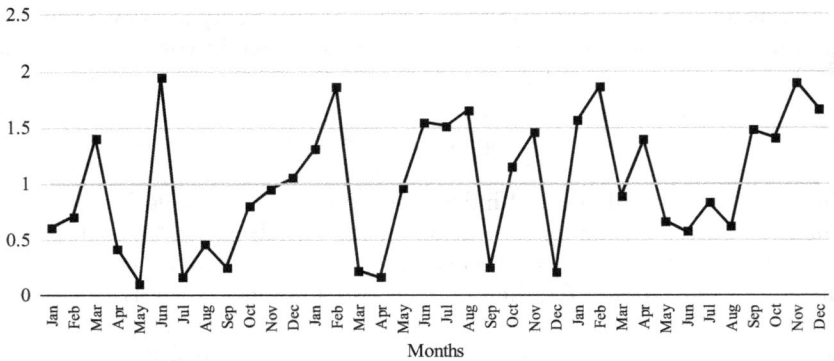

Figure 4.7 Run chart for mortality index.

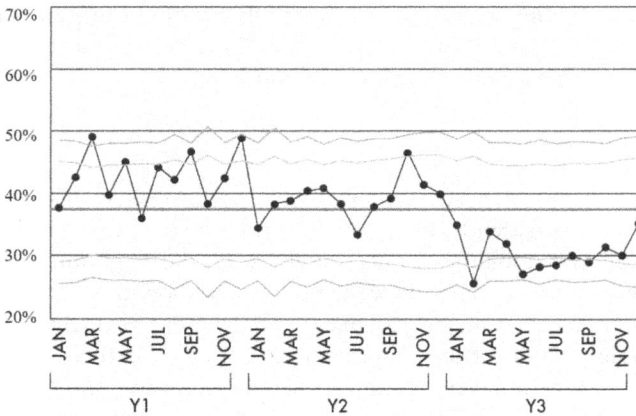

Figure 4.8 Control chart for mortality rate.

Let's interpret an example using severe sepsis mortality. Available outcome metrics are a risk-adjusted mortality index (Figure 4.7), an observed mortality rate (Figure 4.8), a fluid compliance measure for 30 ml/kg (Figure 4.9), and antibiotics compliance within 3 hours (Figure 4.10). The risk-adjusted index provides a story about how the hospital is performing while risk adjusting for variables that impact the mortality. The observed rate provides information to the hospital regarding the performance of that hospital. How does focusing on outcome metrics help drive future improvement initiatives? From a high-level perspective, the observed mortality rate and risk-adjusted mortality index highlight whether or not severe sepsis mortality needs to be improved based on analyzing the data. For example, knowing a 13% mortality rate is equal to a 1.5 risk-adjusted index means that more

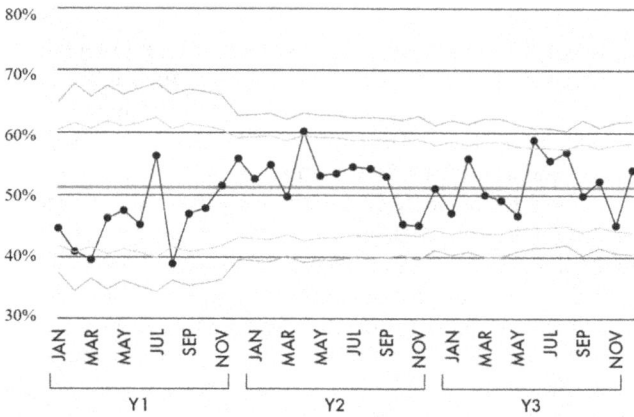

Figure 4.9 Control chart for fluid compliance of 30 ml/kg.

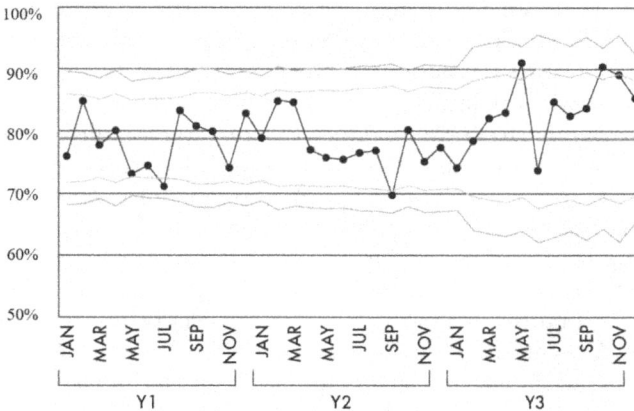

Figure 4.10 Control chart for antibiotic administration within 3 hours.

patients are dying than expected. These two pieces of information could provide insight into how to set a goal. Likewise, if a 13% mortality rate was a 0.4 index, this means that this hospital is performing better than expected. Understanding the relationship between an observed mortality rate and an expected mortality index may lead to different questions. In the first scenario, a 13% mortality rate is not ideal as the equivalent index is 1.5, which means that given the risk-adjusted variables more patients are dying than expected. In the second scenario, a 13% mortality rate is equivalent to a 0.4 index, which means that given the severity of your patients, you are doing well. It might even prompt you to ask the question, "I wonder what the top 10% of performers are doing?" You may also be asking about different metrics that influence mortality, which means you're thinking beyond the outcome metrics provided!

A structured approach to data analysis provides a step-by-step approach to ensure you don't skip over the important pieces. Knowing the outcome metric is helpful, but not the full story. There are many process metrics that influence this sepsis mortality outcome metric. Two of many process variables that impact sepsis mortality are antibiotics and fluid administration. There are many steps in the process to administer antibiotics and fluids, such as the clinician ordering the treatment, pharmacy processing the medication, delivery of the medication or fluids to the clinician starting treatment. Measuring all of these individual processes provides an opportunity to analyze and interpret opportunities to improve if it's determined that time is a critical factor in reducing mortality. Some of these process metrics could be defined as the average time to antibiotic administration, average time to administer fluids, average amount of fluids given based on the patient's weight, etc. Integrating these process and outcome metrics together tells more of a complete story than any individual metric alone.

Monitoring and improving change is effective with the right tools. Statistics should generate as many questions as it does answers. Use this story as a guide to approach change and focus on the FACTS. Think about what happens when change is implemented. Is it easier to change a process or change an outcome? Can you fix an outcome without a process? Can you fix a process with an unknown outcome? Measuring processes is crucial to improving outcomes. It may be easier to say "reduce severe sepsis mortality," but reducing it without changing a process may not impact the outcome. Tools exist to guide thinking towards understanding what process metrics impact outcome metrics. Two methodological approaches to analyze processes are root cause analyses (RCA) and rapid plan–do–study–act (PDSA) cycles. RCA is a methodological process for drilling down to the root cause of why an event happened by continually asking the question "why?" until it is no longer possible to ask why. The rapid PDSA cycle is similar to the scientific method and is a cyclical process for conducting research/performance improvement change quickly. A key to successful improvement is breaking down outcome metrics into processes using process maps/swim lane diagrams available within improvement science methodology to better understand what processes may need to be improved to impact the outcome.

When faced with many outcomes and processes to improve, a question is: where should we focus efforts on change? While this is a loaded question, there are a variety of areas to focus on for making decisions. It is beneficial to review governmental initiatives that impact financial reimbursement as a start for where to focus, such as VBP, bundled payments, or P4P, etc. (see Chapter 7). Other initiatives that impact public perceptions through presenting individual hospital performance (i.e., CMS Star Rating is in Chapter 8) are other alternatives. The one point to consider is that one metric can impact a variety of outcomes. For example, PSI-90 has implications for public perceptions of a hospital's performance and financial implications on other governmental initiatives. Regardless of the decision on where you focus, the main point is to leverage the power of statistics through graphically (i.e., run or control charts) presenting both outcome and process metrics to tell a story.

Discussion Questions

- How do government/organizational initiatives/programs alter your improvement efforts?
- How do you view the relationship between process and outcome metrics?
- If you had to argue over whether or not a control chart is appropriate for outcome metrics, what points would you consider?
- As a healthcare professional reviewing control charts, what are the benefits of focusing on common cause variation as opposed to only special cause?
- What are barriers to implementing change using a process vs. outcome metric?

5 Patient Experience

"Patient experience is a second chance to make a first impression."

Introduction

Think back to any time from the 1970s to today and count how many hospitals have been advertised on TV. Are there more advertisements today compared to many years ago? Why or why not? Is there more heightened awareness with healthcare issues in general? Regardless of the reason, hospitals are competing for market share and financial resources, so transitioning from stand-alone hospitals to seeking out other hospitals to form health organizations is commonplace. Another subtle change is the transition of hospitals from a place where a patient goes to receive care to a place where a patient chooses care based on what they desire (i.e., high-quality service, reputation, outcomes, specific providers, etc.). From a patient perspective, the high-quality service is a three-pronged approach: safety to keep me safe, quality to heal me, and patient experience to be nice to me (Bergomi, 2014; Small & Small, 2011). With respect to customer experience, many organizations outside healthcare could be considered leaders in their respective industries. With more healthcare organizations focusing on the patient experience and quality of service provided, it may be beneficial to emulate best practices on service excellence from organizations outside healthcare (i.e., Disney, Google, Apple, Amazon, etc.). Reflect on your own healthcare experience and ask yourself, why do you stay with your current physician or go to a specific hospital? Or even what stores do you choose to buy clothes at or what restaurants do you eat at? Do you choose to receive care from an organization based on their reputation, quality of care, or the way they treat you?

The reputation of a hospital is vital to retain current patients and attract new ones. Hospitals provide a service and patients expect high-quality service and care. The challenge with providing high-quality service is understanding how patients define (construct validity) high-quality service. The journey down this path requires two components: (1) a clinical expert; and (2) a methodological/statistical expert. Without both types of expertise the end result may be a clinical tool with no validity or a valid tool with no clinical applicability. Over the years, there have been a variety of tools for measuring quality of service or patient experience, with the most common being Consumer Assessment of Healthcare Providers and

Systems (CAHPS), which was created and trademarked by Agency for Healthcare Research and Quality (AHRQ). Collecting this data is a priority for Centers for Medicare/Medicaid Services (CMS) and is tied to financial and performance metrics. AHRQ has a certification process to be a vendor for administering CAHPS that is maintained through National Committee for Quality Assurance (NCQA). It is recommended to select a vendor for administration of CAPHS to ensure credibility and anonymity.

Press Ganey

Press Ganey is one of many approved vendors for measuring patient experience. The history of Press Ganey demonstrates the imagination that one question can accomplish, "Does the way in which cultures around the globe treat health, illness, and healing have any relevance to contemporary medicine?" (www.pressganey. com/about/history-mission). Back in the 1970s Dr. Press asked this question to students and this led him to become an expert in patient satisfaction. Could this be the start of an evolution for evaluating patient experience in a hospital? He had the clinical knowledge, but knew that one piece of information was lacking. In 1984, he realized he was missing a systematic way to both measure (construct validity) and improve patient satisfaction (process metrics to drive outcome). This is where Dr. Ganey became involved as a statistician and methodologist; resulting in the creation of Press Ganey. The relevance behind this story from the 1970s and 1980s is that healthcare professionals in combination with methodologists and statisticians are working together to advance healthcare.

Multiple patient satisfaction surveys have been developed to assess various domains across different places of delivering care. Whether a patient receives services in a hospital, ambulatory center, physician office, nursing home, or emergency department, a survey exists that allows patients to evaluate the place they received care. These results are integral to improvement as there is competition to be the number one performer. Additionally, the structure of healthcare delivery is changing at a rapid pace, such as the rise of urgent care centers, shift of hospital-based care to ambulatory services, government financial initiatives on the entire continuum of care, hospitals reimbursed based on quality of care, individual hospitals merging to become larger health systems, and hospitals seeking other opportunities (i.e., insurance companies, healthcare products, joint ventures, etc.) to generate income. Patients have many choices/opportunities to receive care, so why *choose* you?

Patient Experience

Think about the reasons why you shop in a certain store or why you travel to specific destinations over and over. Is it due to the way you were treated? Is it the destination? Is it the atmosphere? Healthcare is no different. Life is a journey, not a destination, and healthcare professionals are part of the journey through life. As the public gets more technologically savvy, more people will research the best place to receive care based on a hospital's performance for specific outcomes. This research comes from a variety of sources, such as word of mouth, printed/digital advertisements, and/or the internet. Regardless of the validity of the information a patient *chooses* to hear, when patients have the option to choose where to receive care they may focus on the "best" care. Countless advertisements exist to evaluate the best hospital and different grades/stars a hospital receives, like U.S. News, World Report, Leapfrog, Health Insight, Consumer Reports, Star Ratings, etc.

So why is it important to focus on patient experience as opposed to clinical outcomes? Shouldn't hospitals be judged based on a patient's outcome instead of the patient's experience in a hospital? The answer is that a multitude of factors are associated with clinical outcomes. Patient experience is one of those factors and appears in other analyses (i.e., CMS provides publicly available data to compare performance). Two sources provided by CMS are the Star Rating and Hospital Compare. CMS Star Rating (Chapter 8) ranks hospital performance on a variety of indicators, culminating in assigning 1–5 stars. CMS Hospital Compare (Chapter 9) provides individual measures for comparing performance on up to three hospitals. The implication is that CMS initiatives tie financial compensation and performance to patient experience measures utilizing Hospital Consumer Assessment of Healthcare Providers and Systems (HCAHPS) as a measure for overall hospital performance.

A study analyzing risk-adjusted data using CMS Hospital Compare found a statistically significant relationship that patient experience was related to more favorable clinical outcomes, which provides support for the inclusion of patient experience data in how hospitals are reimbursed for services (Trzeciak, Gaughan, Bosire, & Mazzarelli, 2016). Despite this positive finding, Manary, Boulding, Staelin, and Glickman (2013) expressed three concerns regarding the use of patient experience measures and their influence on outcomes: (1) patient satisfaction captures happiness, which is influenced by factors not related to medical treatment; (2) patient experience measures are confounded by factors not associated with process or quality; and (3) patient experience is based on a clinician fulfilling a patient's need to receive a desired treatment. The drive to earn high scores on patient experience has the potential to lead to "bad medicine" (Junewicz & Youngner, 2015). The counterargument is that patient experience is a complex variable to measure. A valid and reliable measure for patient experience will capture the complexity of the construct and be more representative of the entire patient experience.

Regardless of your views, patient experience data has made its way into performance metrics and financial reimbursement. Patients are more educated regarding the care they receive and have expectations on how they receive care. Patient experience surveys afford patients a voice to evaluate their experience with a healthcare organization. Understanding the impact and how to improve patient satisfaction scores becomes critical for future success and retention of patients. The bigger question is, how to leverage patient experience data to drive improvement? It's easy to jump to conclusions about what could be done. Start from the beginning. Take a step back and think methodologically about how patient experience is defined. Patient experience is a complex variable that cannot be directly observed or measured, which in research methodology is referred to as a **latent variable**. Another example of a latent variable is measuring an individual's intelligence quotient (IQ). An individual's IQ consists of measurable traits, such as mathematical, spatial, verbal, etc. that are directly observed and measured.

Patient experience means different things to different people and patient satisfaction is one aspect (Bleich, Özaltin, & Murray, 2009). All of these varied definitions relate to a component of how patient experience is measured. Knowing how patients perceive their experience begins with asking them. The first step in the process of understanding constructs is to methodologically approach how they are operationalized or defined (construct validity). These measures are often statistically analyzed as **percentile ranks**. As a healthcare professional, being faced with improving percentile ranks is complicated and a struggle to accomplish as it is difficult to predict and modify human behavior. There are no rules or laws of human behavior and predicting with 100% accuracy how everyone will respond is not possible or a one-size-fits-all approach is not effective. Psychology experts have developed many theories for understanding how to influence human behavior, but it will not work 100% of the time. As a result, it is not surprising to hear from healthcare professionals that an intervention may work for one type of patient, but not another. While an intervention is not expected to solve every type of situation, a methodological approach to breaking down the healthcare delivery process is the best approach to critically evaluate how patients view their experience to develop solutions.

Behaviors and State of Mind

Patient satisfaction is one aspect of patient experience and is no different than mortality or readmission measures or infection indices. Break down the healthcare delivery process that a patient receives into process and outcome metrics. Any potential interaction between a healthcare professional and patient has the ability to influence a patient's perception of their experience. As Maya Angelou said, "I've learned that people will forget what you said, people will forget what you did, but people will never forget how you made them feel." These interactions may leave a temporary or permanent memory for that patient to reflect on when completing their patient experience survey. A behavior may have a longer-lasting impression/impact on a patient; whereas some events may result in temporarily impacting a patient's state of mind. Is it possible that a phenomenal experience outweighs a negative experience? What are the factors that drive patients to respond in specific ways?

Leveraging this thought, behaviors and state of mind are two powerful concepts when developing interventions. Translating behaviors and state of mind concepts into practice is the same process as defining process and outcome metrics. How does patient satisfaction relate to behaviors? Is satisfaction a behavior or a state of mind? In other words, will patients with a bad experience in the emergency department rate the rest of their hospital stay favorably? Or could a patient with a bad experience with one healthcare professional and an exceptional experience with another healthcare professional rate his/her experience favorably?

Determining factors influencing positive perceptions of patient experience is critical. The objective is to know whether to influence a state of mind or a behavior. Often times the initial reaction to a bad experience is to solve the problem and move on. While this is appropriate, understanding behaviorally why an experience was bad is the start of developing an intervention to improve. As an example, during an interview for an employee engagement specialist at a hospital seeking to develop interventions around improving patient satisfaction, one of many questions revolved around "how do you convince a pharmacist with no patient contact that he/she can impact patient satisfaction?" Considering an answer to this question requires a methodological approach and not a gut reaction. "Because it does" is not an effective response. Think about the process of what occurs within a hospital. A pharmacist with no direct patient contact has indirect contact with patients through interactions with nursing staff who care for patients. A pharmacist's negative behavior on the phone can translate into altering a nurse's state of mind to cause a temporary change in mood, which makes its way back to the patient. This mood change may resolve within a few minutes/ hours, but the pharmacist's behavior may continue. Fixing the problem stems from understanding the processes impacting the outcome.

Behavior change is complex. The focus may begin with things within an individual's control. For example, a floor nurse organizes their time to administer patient medications, but has less control over ensuring radiology comes at the scheduled time. Knowing any interaction with a patient impacts the patient's experience creates a need to ensure healthcare professionals consistently (reliability) exhibit desirable behaviors. In this example, perhaps open direct communication could help manage patient expectations.

Our goal is to motivate employees to engage in a behavior to maximize results or improve the patient experience. Many motivation theories exist to engage and motivate the workforce. Some popular theories are Maslow's hierarchy of needs, equity theory, expectancy theory, reinforcement theory, and work design theory (Muchinsky, 2006). Within healthcare, goal-setting theory and self-regulation theory are considered motivation theories and provide techniques to drive improvement and accountability to not only engage a team but improve satisfaction. Does an engaged workforce equal a satisfied patient? Or does a satisfied patient equal an engaged employee? The National Alliance for Quality Care released a white paper on why patient and family engagement is critical for nursing (www.naqc.org/WhitePaper-PatientEngagement).

To begin to understand the relationship between satisfaction and engagement, leverage the skills learned and think about what questions to ask. How do patients define satisfaction? How are experience, satisfaction, and engagement defined? How do they impact patient outcomes? Is it possible that satisfaction could be a state of mind? Can patients be both satisfied and dissatisfied and what impact does this have on patient experience? How easily can someone move from satisfaction to dissatisfaction, or vice versa? Is engagement a behavior? Is it possible to go from being engaged to disengaged or vice versa?

During one lecture on satisfaction and engagement the take-home message was that engagement was a buzz word for satisfaction. As a result, satisfaction and engagement were used interchangeably throughout the lecture as they were determined to be related. While there is some truth to that, the underlying drivers differ. The presenter was engaging, but the lecture wasn't satisfying. Simply being engaged is not a sufficient condition for satisfaction (remember reliability is a necessary, but not sufficient, condition for validity). The idea that satisfaction and engagement are closely related has been studied frequently, where one study shows strong, positive correlations between engagement and satisfaction. However, these correlations are likely due to semantic similarities between engagement and satisfaction (Nimon, Shuck, & Zigarmi, 2016). Another explanation is engagement and satisfaction measure a higher-level latent variable (i.e., a variable that cannot be directly observed or measured) called patient experience, so satisfaction and engagement are two variables that measure a higher variable called patient experience. Despite similar results, how measures are defined is important to understand the interpretation.

The question remains, is satisfaction an attitude or state of mind and is engagement a behavior? Debating the differences between satisfaction and engagement is not as important as developing interventions that impact both satisfaction and engagement. The question is, what to focus on first? Satisfaction or engagement? Does a satisfied patient lead to a more engaged employee? Does an engaged patient mean that they are more satisfied? Focus on the construct that has the largest impact. Understanding the link between engagement and how it relates to satisfaction sheds light on how to improve behavior to increase patient satisfaction. A patient's satisfaction can change in an instant as a result of a healthcare provider's behavior. The only way to know how patients feel about their experience is as simple as asking them.

Survey Methodology

Multiple measures exist for evaluating patient experience, with one commonly used survey being CAHPS. CAHPS surveys are available for hospitals, home health, fee-for-service, Medicare advantage and prescription drug plan, in-center hemodialysis, nationwide adult Medicaid, hospice, accountable care organizations participating in Medicare initiatives, outpatient and ambulatory surgery, Physician Quality Reporting System (PQRS), Merit-Based Incentive Payment System (MIPS), and the emergency department. These statistics provide valuable insight into decision making and breaking down the statistical concepts generates questions. From a methodological perspective, HCAHPS utilizes 27 questions over 10 patient satisfaction domains for inpatient and outpatient services.

Many healthcare professionals opt to do survey research, because the perception is that survey research is easier to conduct. This couldn't be further from the truth; developing a survey is challenging and takes tremendous knowledge and skill to ensure the survey is reliable and valid. Dillman (2007) is an expert in the field of survey methodology and has written many books on the topic. The generic development of a survey involves survey questions and response scales. The nuances of the development of these two components to a survey are complex.

Researchers have demonstrated that the type of question and response scale can influence responses.

Survey Questions

Survey questions are written in a variety of formats, ranging from the type of question (i.e., measures related to attitudes, beliefs, or fact-based questions) to the structure of the question (i.e., open vs. closed-ended questions). The basic premise behind any survey question is it must be clear and answerable for any person responding to the question. Dillman (2007) posed a simple question, "about how many cups of coffee do you drink a day?" This question creates many challenges and is not as straightforward as it may appear.

1. How many ounces define a cup?
2. A person who doesn't drink coffee can't answer this question.
3. If a person provides a 0, then does this indicate that he/she is not a coffee drinker or didn't drink coffee on the day in question?
4. What is the time reference to this question? Is it today only? Or is it generalizing to a daily average over the course of a week or month?

The other issue is the structure of the question. Open-ended questions allow for written responses. The advantage is a person may write about something that wasn't thought of when writing a question. The disadvantage is written responses are qualitative. Qualitative analyses take time to analyze. Closed-ended questions require individuals to rate on a response scale. The advantage is a structured analysis. The disadvantage is responses elicited from closed-ended questions are limited to the phrasing of the question. Notice the advantages and disadvantages are reversed between closed-ended vs. open-ended questions. Open-ended are harder to analyze, but provide insight into issues not thought about. Closed-ended are easier to analyze, but limit issues to how questions are defined.

Response Scales

The response scale selected for rating a question is equally as important as the writing of the question. Not only does the question phrasing influence a response, but the measurement scale selected influences question responses. As discussed in Chapter 2, response scales are related to scales of measurement. Nominal and ordinal scales are qualitative and interval and ratio scales are quantitative. The scale of measurement selected dictates the statistical analysis. One common response scale in surveys is the Likert scale, which was developed by Likert (1932). A Likert scale consists of usually 5 or 7 points to rate questions designed as a **unipolar** or **bipolar scale**.

Unipolar or bipolar scales are the most common format for labeling rating scales. A unipolar scale measures one aspect of a behavior and a bipolar scale is designed to capture both aspects of a behavior. For example, a unipolar scale measuring satisfaction may only focus on variations in levels of satisfaction and not

Table 5.1 Unipolar and bipolar scales

Scale type	1	2	3	4	5
Unipolar	Not at all satisfied	Slightly satisfied	Moderately satisfied	Satisfied	Extremely satisfied
Bipolar	Extremely dissatisfied	Dissatisfied	Neither dissatisfied nor satisfied	Satisfied	Extremely satisfied

dissatisfaction, so the scale would be from not at all satisfied to extremely satisfied. A bipolar scale focuses on measuring levels of dissatisfaction and satisfaction, so a scale would be from extremely unsatisfied to extremely satisfied. The advantage of a unipolar scale is examining greater variability in responses to one side of the scale, because on a 5-point scale only the first point is not at all satisfied and the other four are variations in satisfaction. A bipolar scale has limited responses for both satisfaction and dissatisfaction, so that on a 5-point scale there are likely two responses for dissatisfaction and two for satisfaction. Either response scale is appropriate for survey development. See Table 5.1 for an example of unipolar and bipolar scale.

HCAHPS Survey

The HCAHPS survey is used by hospitals and was developed in 2002 when CMS collaborated with AHRQ to develop the survey. Endorsed by the National Quality Forum (NQF) in 2005, HCAHPS is publicly available for reporting purposes (i.e., performance and financial). The HCAHPS survey consists of 27 questions over 10 domains that assess a patient's hospital experience. The domains assessed are: communication with nurses, communication with doctors, responsiveness of hospital staff, pain management, communication about medicines, discharge information, cleanliness of hospital environment, quietness of hospital environment, overall rating of hospital, and willingness to recommend hospital. Patients are randomly selected to participate in the survey via telephone or paper 48 hours to 6 weeks after being discharged. To ensure the validity of the responses, CMS engages in quality control of responses and adjusts based on factors deemed beyond the hospital's control.

Knowing the domains and number of questions is important, but reflecting on methodological questions provides a frame of reference for what further information is needed prior to the analysis. Some questions include: what is the **response rate** of the survey? What are the inclusion and exclusion criteria for being selected to take the survey? Are there benchmarks to compare performance? Is the whole population surveyed or a sample? How was the sample selected? How are responses deemed valid? When is the data finalized? Answering these questions provides greater clarity with understanding the methodology of the sample responses and creates objectivity to focus on the facts of the analysis.

An important factor in driving change starts with understanding the content of the questions being asked. For example, there's a global question asking about the patient's willingness to recommend the hospital. From a methodological perspective, what is the patient thinking about when they read the word "recommend." Not knowing how patients answer this question makes it challenging to develop an intervention to improve. Perhaps the patient is being primed based on questions before or after this question or maybe they are thinking about an interaction with a healthcare professional or experience with a particular department. Any of these explanations is plausible. The only way to really know what a patient is recommending is to ask him or her. Before asking questions, it's important to understand how the metric is operationalized. Depending on the metric being measured, the inclusion/exclusion criteria may be conceptually opposite from each other. Utilize the DEFINE tool to understand what calculations are included in the willingness to recommend score.

- Denominator – all patients responding to the survey.
- Exclusion criteria – patients < 18 years old, length of stay < 1 day, psychiatric patients, patients with foreign addresses, and the following dispositions: expirations, nursing homes, hospice, skilled nursing facilities, and court/law enforcement.
- Factor – scores are converted to a top/bottom-box percentage where ratings of 9 or 10 are top-box and ratings less than 6 are bottom-box.
- Inclusion criteria – patients ≥ 18 years old, length of stay > 1 day, patients discharged alive.
- Numerator – patients rating 9 or 10 for top-box and 6 or below for bottom-box.
- Evaluate – metric is based on a score calculated as either a top/bottom-box score. This is *not* a percentile, but can be converted. Evaluation of positive/negative perceptions.

Statistical Method Review

The next methodological approach to analyzing HCAHPS data is defining the available statistical concepts. The calculated statistics are response rates, sample size, percentile rank, overall score, and top/bottom-box score. Individual statistics provide one side of the story, but a combination of many statistics tells the whole story. Use your insight by focusing on the FACTS to understand the statistics presented to generate questions.

One question posed earlier was related to the response rate of the sample. This statistic is calculated by the total number of patients responding to the survey divided by the total number of surveys sent. If this is not provided, then request it. While HCAPHS samples the population, some healthcare organizations survey the entire population. The implication of a response rate provides insight as to whether or not the results generalize from the sample to the entire population (i.e., external validity). Lower response rates impact the variability of the results. Smaller sample sizes have larger standard deviations and larger samples have smaller standard deviations. An average score from a larger sample may be closer to the population average.

With respect to response rates, there are two initial issues. The first issue is that the average survey response rate for published studies is around 34% (Fulton, 2018). Kaplowitz, Hadlock, and Levine (2004) studied differences between mail and internet survey response rates with various points of contact using Dillman's (2007) method to improve response rates. The response rates utilizing under-graduate students ranged from 28.6% to 31.5% (Kaplowitz et al., 2004). Cook, Heath, and Thompson (2000) conducted a meta-analysis of 68 surveys within 49 studies utilizing mail and internet-based surveys with varying degrees of con-tact (i.e., pre-survey letter, thank you postcard, etc.). They found the average response rate was 39.6% with a standard deviation of 19.6%. One key driver to increasing response rates is a double-edged sword and that is a follow-up reminder. While follow-up reminders have been shown to improve response rates, too many reminders result in a decrease in response rates. Surveys with no follow-up reminder at all ranged between 25% and 30%. In conclusion, response rates to surveys vary between 20% and 30% with the potential of utilizing multiple points of contact to improve rates (Cook et al., 2000).

The second issue is the differences between individuals responding to the survey compared to those who did not. This is referred to as **non-response bias**. Armstrong and Overton (1977) noted issues with mail surveys and the impact of non-response bias. Being able to estimate non-response bias is important to gen-eralize sample results to the population to make improvement decisions. Barclay, Todd, Finlay, Grande, and Wyatt (2002) examined methods to improve response rates, predict non-response, and assess non-response bias in mail surveys. They found differences in sample results compared to non-response and suggest the importance of sending at least three reminders to healthcare professionals to reduce non-response.

To draw conclusions from survey results requires a sample of data representative of the population. Knowing it is not possible to always get 100% of the popula-tion, representative random sample is selected to generalize results to the popula-tion. Response rates and the issue of non-response bias compromise the validity of the results. Improving response rates through multiple points of contact (i.e., follow-up reminders) improves the sample size at the same time as reducing the non-response bias. This is important, because HCAHPS requires a minimum of 300 randomly sampled responses over a 12-month period to send CMS results. A defined methodology to improve response rates is beneficial to the quality of the results. Randomly selecting patients through a probability sampling technique protects the integrity of the process and ensures all patients have an equal chance of being selected. This combined methodology results in the greater likelihood of the sample representing the population.

The next statistic is the percentile rank, which is a complex calculation with tremendous value for interpretation. Recall from Chapter 3 that percentile ranks are statistical measures used for comparative purposes to determine how a healthcare organization scores in relation to others. As an example, a hospital in the 63rd percentile is doing better than 63% of the other organizations or 37% of organizations are doing better than you. The percentile rank is important for two reasons: (1) it compares performance to others; and (2) percentile ranks are calculated using overall scores.

Comparative performance provides insight into how an organization performs in relation to the rest of the organizations included in the dataset. If possible, knowing the 25th, 50th, and 75th percentile rank and score provides more information, but is not always available. The 50th percentile provides a frame of reference as to an individual hospital's location among a larger dataset where half the organizations are above that score and the other half are below. Statistically, percentiles form a standard normal distribution or bell-shaped curve. Movement between percentiles is easier in the middle of the distribution and more challenging on the extremes of the distribution. In other words, it is easier for organizations to move between the 25th and 75th percentiles than move between the 1st and 10th or 90th and 99th percentiles.

From a methodological perspective, a percentile rank is derived from an overall score tied to the individual patient rating. HCAHPS is a 5-point Likert-type scale from 1 to 5 where the numbers are converted to a score of 0–100. A rating of 1 is equivalent to 0, 2 is equal to 25, 3 is equal to 50, 4 is equal to 75, and 5 is equal to 100. The overall score is calculated by summing all the scored responses and dividing by a count of responses received. Testing your creativity with the statistics allows for leveraging your skills to ask questions regarding the statistics. For example, if an overall score is 81.3, then anything less than a rating of 5 results in a decrease in the overall score, because a 4 is equal to a 75. Knowing the sample size sheds light on how much influence one individual response has on the overall score. For simplicity purposes, if there are four responses with three rating a 5 and one rating a 1, then the average would be 75 (100 + 100 + 100 + 0 divided by 4). This same example, with 40 responses with 39 rating a 5 and one rating a 1, would result in a mean of 97.5. Mathematically, the more responses, the less influence on the overall score. Thus, how many responses are included in the overall score becomes important. For reimbursement purposes, CMS may have a defined quota of monthly responses to ensure consistency and mitigate potential mathematical influences on scores where all hospitals are treated the same. Hypothetically, if a random sample of 200 discharges a month is set, then questions relate to the external validity of the 200 sample for hospitals that may have 1,000 monthly discharges to another hospital that may have 10,000 monthly discharges. Decisions must be made either way, so knowledge of the methodology behind the decisions is critical.

The final statistic of top/bottom-box score is vital for comparative purposes. Similar to the percentile rank, the top/bottom-box score is calculated on the basis of the top and bottom scores selected for a particular question. The top-box score is calculated based on the best possible response that is selected by patients, which is generally a response of "always," "definitely yes," a rating of 9 or 10, "strongly agree." The bottom-box score is calculated based on "sometimes or never," "definitely no," a rating of 6 or lower, "strongly disagree," or "disagree." Since questions are rated using different rating scales, the purpose of categorizing into a top/bottom-box score is to calculate a universal percentage that applies to all questions. This percentage is then used for calculating percentiles for comparative purposes. There is one caveat to the interpretation of percentiles for the top/bottom-box.

Normally, the higher percentile indicates better performance, which is true for the top-box score. This means that scoring in the 95th percentile for the top-box represents performance better than 95% of other organizations. The calculation of percentiles is based on the percentage of patients who respond favorably to the survey items. For example, a rating of 9 or 10 is used to calculate the top-box, so a higher score indicates more patients viewed the organization in a favorable manner. The rationale is a higher individual rating score on the 5-point Likert-type scale equates to a higher positive perception based on how the questions are answered.

The opposite is true for the bottom-box score. This calculation is based on negative perceptions of the organization, so a lower score is more desirable. Using the same example, patients rating a 6 or lower are calculated in the bottom-box score, so a higher percentage indicates more patients viewed their experience as less favorable. In other words, if the bottom-box score was 70%, then this would mean that 70% of patients responding to the survey rated their experience a 6 or less. Conversely, the remaining 30% gave a rating above 6. The corresponding percentiles are based on low to high scores, which means the 10th percentile indicates lower negative perceptions of a patient's experience and the 90th percentile indicates higher negative perceptions.

Results

Whatever vendor is used for administering HCAHPS likely results in providing multiple options/graphs for obtaining HCAHPS data, but downloading raw data provides the greatest flexibility for an analysis. Statistics available for download include: percentile ranks, observed scores, benchmark comparisons with percentile ranks and scores, and sample sizes. Integrating multiple statistics generates insights into the data to tell a complete story analytically and drive future questions. Thinking methodologically about how the metrics and samples are defined tests your creativity to understand the data statistically and allows for an objective critical analysis of the results. The creativity of how the data is best visualized to tell the story is limited to what you can think of. Focusing on only the percentile rank will only tell one piece of a larger story. A percentile rank message could be: "your unit needs to improve its 23rd percentile rank." Multiple statistics combined together provide a more complete picture of what is happening in an effort to focus improvement initiatives and drive change. Focus on the FACTS of the results being presented to remove subjectivity and provide an objective analysis.

Creating Graphs

There are many ways of storytelling with data, but an effective method is one that generates more questions than answers. One way to use the insight learned from experience is to leverage various statistics to create a cohesive story. A graphical representation of statistics provides an easy-to-understand visual of the data.

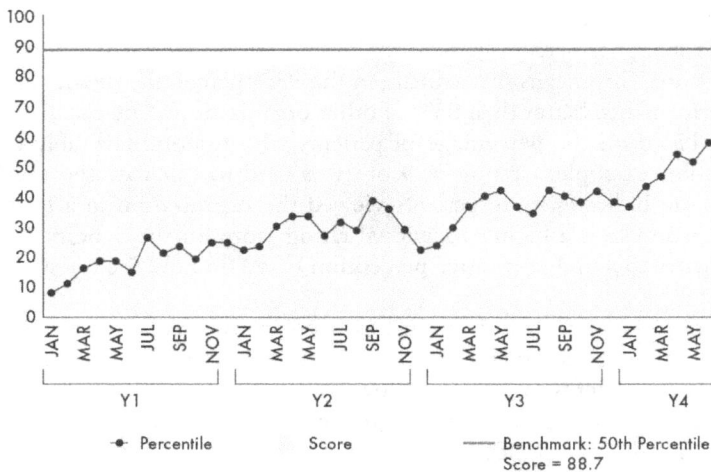

Figure 5.1 Hospital Consumer Assessment of Healthcare Providers and Systems (HCAHPS) question analysis.

Run/control charts were one effective graphical display to trend data over time. Overall, there are many decisions/choices for graphically displaying data to achieve effective results. For the purposes of this visualization, the percentile rank was created as a run chart without the inclusion of an overall mean (Figure 5.1). The mean could be added, but in this case an average comparison may not be ideal considering the average score to achieve the 50th percentile is included. Too many statistics can create information overload and take away from the purpose of the graph. Sometimes simpler is better! Regardless of an average being present or not, the run chart monitors trends over time to determine increasing or decreasing trends within the data. You can also use the run chart rules to identify patterns/trends. Percentile ranks allow comparisons between an individual hospital in relation to the entire database. The bar in the background of Figure 5.1 represents the monthly score that corresponds to the monthly percentile rank. In addition to the score and rank for this individual hospital, the 50th percentile rank and score for the entire database are displayed on the graph with a dotted line.

Think methodologically before interpreting the results by focusing on the FACTS.

- Formulas – average score comprised of the sum of the values divided by the count of the responses. Each rating that makes up the score is converted to a value of 0, 25, 50, 75, or 100 that corresponds to a rating of 1, 2, 3, 4, or 5, respectively. The percentile rank is a comparative value that converts the raw score to a percentile for comparative purposes.
- Analyze patterns/trends – monthly percentile rank is slowly trending up with some variability. Average score is hovering around the 50th percentile score.

- Consider guidelines/rules – run chart rules for interpretation apply. Statistical rules indicate that the percentile rank is comprised of an overall score, which is related to an individual ranking.
- Think – the 50th percentile rank is equivalent to an 89.3 score. A rating of 4 is equivalent to a score of 75 and a rating of 5 is equivalent to 100. This indicates that improving the percentile rank involves improving a patient's score from a 4 to a 5. An observed score of 88.0 to 88.4 (any value 88.5 or above rounds to 89) ranges from the 29th to 37th percentile. This demonstrates a wide range of percentiles for minor changes in a 0.1 increase in an overall score when scores are around the mean.
- Statistics – percentile rank and average score.

With the FACTS presented, take time to think about the implications from a methodological perspective. The formulas and guidelines/rules for the calculation of the percentile rank indicate results are comprised of scores translating into individual ratings where a survey rating of 1 equates to a score of 0, a 2 is 25, a 3 is 50, a 4 is 75, and a 5 is 100. Focus on two particular months where Mar Y4 has a percentile rank of 45 and May Y4 has a percentile rank of 49. Both of these ranks correspond to a score of 89 and some 0.1 value. This could be 89.2 and 89.4 or any other combination from 88.5 to 89.4, which would all round to 89. What matters is not what value corresponds to a tenth of a decimal point, but rather that a small change can span a variety of percentile ranks for scores if the score is around the mean.

Percentiles are standardized, which makes the interpretation similar to z-scores on a bell-shaped curve. See Figure 5.2 for a visual display of percentiles and standard deviations compared to the bell-shaped curve. While it appears small changes in scores span multiple percentiles, this is true for scores around the mean. Scores on the extremes (i.e., beyond 2 SD) require larger changes to move percentiles. Notice that 1 SD above the mean results in the 50th to 85th percentiles and improving from the 95th percentile to the 99th percentile corresponds to 1SD. The overall conclusion is movement between the 15th and 85th percentiles is more sensitive

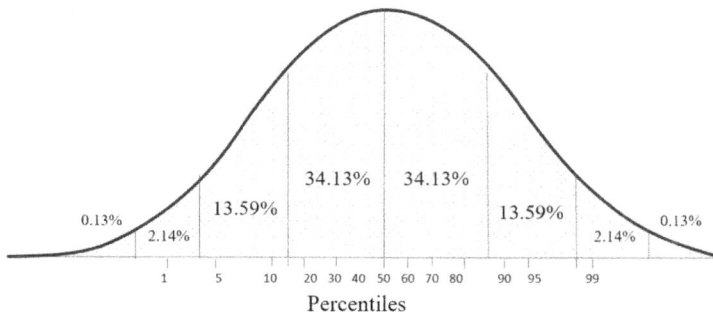

Figure 5.2 Normal distribution comparison to standard deviation and percentiles.

to minor changes in scores compared to moving from the 95th to 99th percentile. Consider the following example of a 50th-percentile score of 88 with a standard deviation of 2. The scores that are 1 SD above the mean range from 88 to 90, which translates to the 50th to 85th percentile. The 95th percentile is 1.5 SD above the mean and the 99th percentile is more than 2 SD from the mean. This translates into a score of 90.5 for the 95th percentile and above a 92 for the 99th percentile. As a result, a 2-point increase in scores around the 50th percentile score spans 36 percentiles (50th to 85th), whereas a 1.5 score increase on the extreme end spans 5 percentiles (95th to 99th).

The overall story objectively interpreted from focusing on the FACTS and reviewing the graph indicates a slight improvement over time. More specifically, variability within the percentile rank increasing and decreasing could lead to variations in the process or a reflection of total responses. Knowing the monthly response rate will indicate how much of an impact that one response has on the overall average. Despite minor variability over time, there is improvement from the beginning of the time period to the end. There is variability within percentile ranks based on an overall score where a small change in an observed score has an impact on the overall percentile rank. In other words, the highest percentile rank is 42, which corresponds to a score of 89. Taking into consideration rounding up for a value of 88.5 to 88.9 and rounding down from 89.1 to 89.4 means that this 42nd percentile rank could result in an observed score from 88.5 to 89.4. Knowing the 50th percentile rank score is 89.3, this eliminates 89.3 and 89.4 as plausible scores. Leveraging the insight gained from the relationship between percentile rank to score to individual rating indicates that a rating of 4 equates to a score of 75 and a rating of 5 equates to 100. Depending on the sample size, the impact of any rating increase (i.e., 1 to 2, 2 to 3, 3 to 4, or 4 to 5) could have the plausibility of increasing an overall score by 0.1 of a point. The magnitude of the impact is contingent on sample size and/or an individual rating of 1–5.

Discussion

Latent variables like human behavior and patient experience are challenging to influence, because developing interventions around variables that cannot be directly measured is complicated. Change may work for one individual, but not another. As a result, it's common to tweak interventions as additional knowledge and experience are gained. An individual's behavior and subsequent experience with an organization have the potential of being influenced by attitudes, beliefs, emotions, and prior experience, so this is the first step to understanding how to initiate change. The intervention begins by defining metrics of interest through understanding how they are measured to develop an intervention that addresses that metric.

Obtaining all the FACTS and methodologically defining the metric provides objective information to tell the story. The next step is how to proceed and take action with the insights gained from the analytics to determine what questions to ask. From a methodological perspective, operationalizing process metrics that improve desired outcomes is the second step. The first aim of the Three Pillars of Statistics is met, which is know your numbers. The remaining question is how to translate the given information into a sustainable behavioral intervention. The last aim, setting goals to drive change, is critical to ensure meaningful and achievable goals are developed beyond someone saying to "increase their percentile rank."

Patient satisfaction is operationalized by the 10 domains within HCAHPS. Defining these domains and understanding how processes impact outcomes is an effective methodology to develop behavioral interventions. Individual variables precede the development of process/outcome metrics, so understanding how patient experience variables are defined by patients helps to focus improvement efforts. All individuals are motivated by different factors, which explains why some interventions work for some people and not for others. To better understand variables that influence a patient's experience is to conduct a focus group. Improving a process without understanding others' perception may not lead to the desired improvement.

For example, when developing questions to ask patients regarding the likelihood to recommend questions, it's plausible to ask patients if they are influenced by: (1) items before the likelihood to recommend question; (2) an overwhelming positive or negative experience within the hospital; (3) the reputation of the organization; and (4) their willingness to recommend the organization based on food or cleanliness of the room, etc. Even though some questions are addressed by other questions on the survey, it's easy to jump to conclusions about what patients are recommending, but asking patents directly is more effective to know what is important. This point comes down to the open-ended vs. closed-ended questions. The closed-ended questions mean perceptions are limited to how the survey was designed and open-ended questions allow patients to explicitly state their opinions.

Every patient interaction has two potential outcomes: (1) the interaction leaves a long-lasting impression; or (2) the interaction has a temporary impact on the patient. These two interactions correspond to potential outcomes that impact their behavior for the remainder of the hospital stay or their attitude that has a short impact on their hospital stay. Behaviors and emotions significantly influence how others react in given situations. This reaction may stay with the patient temporarily or be the reason, both positive and negative, for how they respond to the patient experience survey. Consistent delivery of care is critical. Humans are creatures of habit, so incorporating processes into behavioral responses results in consistent and automatic delivery. When a process is not well learned, individuals require conscious decision making to initiate the process, which decreases the chance of adopting change (Ouellette & Wood, 1998).

The third aim of the Three Pillars of Statistics is setting goals to drive change. Goal-setting theory focuses on the development of SMART goals, which effectively drive accountability through appropriately set goals. SMART goals must be specific, measurable, actionable, relevant, and time-bound. Setting an appropriate goal depends on the question being answered. A potential SMART goal could be to improve the likelihood to recommend percentile rank to the 50th percentile within 1 year. One aspect of this goal that must be assessed is whether or not it is a realistic goal.

Setting goals for the sake of being mathematically or methodologically sound may not be ideal. As an example, setting a goal of a 10% increase to be above the 50th percentile for overall patient experience score may not be achievable. If the 50th percentile rank average score is an 80, then a 10% increase is an 88. Knowing a rating of 4 equals 75 and a 5 equals 100 means any patient rating a 4 decreases the score. Minor changes in scores impact percentiles ranging from 15 to 85, but the 0 to 14 and 86th to 99th percentiles are less influenced by small changes. As a result, improving from the 50th to 55th percentile requires a smaller change in score than improving from the 90th to 95th percentile. Sometimes we focus the right efforts on the wrong question. Improving percentile ranks is challenging, but a better approach is refocusing the question from percentile rank to how does a healthcare organization encourage a patient giving a rating of a 5 instead of a 4?

Once a SMART goal is set, the challenge is operationalizing the goal to develop interventions for improvement. Focusing on the FACTS demonstrates the importance of utilizing statistics to tell the story and aid in setting goals. From a methodology perspective, focusing on developing a hypothesis and searching the literature provides insight as to what others are doing and generates potential ideas for interventions. Knowing the ultimate outcome is to improve a patient's likelihood to recommend a hospital means that there are many process metrics that impact the outcome. Defining these process metrics and conducting plan–do–study–act (PDSA) cycles to develop small tests of change aid in refining the process.

The ability to influence human behavior towards positive outcomes is complex considering there are only theories regarding how humans react in given situations. Although the best predictor of future behavior is past behavior, this is only true for behavioral actions that are well learned. Behaviors not well learned or difficult to engage in may be led by intentions, which in turn guide behavior (Ouellette & Wood, 1998). Despite our best efforts for developing sound behavioral interventions, sometimes good intentions lead to different outcomes. Taking a step back and thinking methodologically is an effective approach to drive change.

Patient experience is assessed by the 10 domains of HCAHPS and means different things to different people (Bleich et al., 2009). Using the insights gained, breaking apart concepts into manageable pieces is the beginning step to creating sustainable change. From a methodological perspective, patient experience has been operationalized as patient satisfaction, which is further defined into specific domains that can be measured. The overall constructs of nurse and physician communication, hospital environment, medications, and pain control are a few domains that have been shown to measure patient satisfaction. If the overall outcome is patient experience, then process metrics can be developed that address specific domains. Knowing the complexity of human behavior brings up the issue of how to impact patient satisfaction. Patient experience is here to stay given the emphasis of government initiatives utilizing these metrics for financial and performance incentives.

Discussion Questions

- What value do you see in incorporating a clinical expert and a methodologist/statistician together to innovate healthcare solutions?
- Patients have many choices/opportunities to receive care; why would they choose yours? What service qualities make your organization different?
- What is the value of focusing on the patient experience as opposed to clinical outcomes?
- If you had to define patient experience, what would it look like to you? Is patient experience another word for patient satisfaction? Is it a behavior or state of mind?
- Have you used patient experience data to drive improvement? Were you successful? What did you learn?
- Does an engaged workforce mean a satisfied patient? Can a satisfied patient indicate an engaged employee?
- What are some ways in which you used percentile ranks to drive improvement efforts? How would you change your approach based on what we said?

6 AHRQ Safety Survey

"You can't change what you don't measure, and you can't act on what you don't ask."

Introduction

Knowledge is power and power is knowing how to leverage statistics for effective storytelling to drive change. Statistics are designed to answer questions, determine future direction, and stimulate critical thinking. The challenging aspect of statistics is developing an effective visual display for others to see and understand the story. As individuals, we are all programmed differently where learning styles vary from visual to didactic to hands-on to experiential, and so forth. Knowing your audience by capturing multiple learning techniques into a visual can maximize the effectiveness of your story. Creating graphical representations of data is the most common methodology for presenting statistics, but it's not the only way. The problem with graphical displays is that a picture is worth a thoursand words and not everyone is a visual learner. Anyone can interpret a picture in ways that may generate unintended questions, lead performance improvement down the wrong path, or potentially make others defensive or reactive instead of encouraging an offensive and proactive stance for improvement.

The goal is to transition reactive tendencies towards statistics through building a skill set to objectively interpret data. There will always be individuals poking holes in an analysis or criticizing the validity of the data. Some common criticisms are:

1. Focus on the numbers and look for inconsistencies between graphs.
2. Discuss the color or font sizes of the results.
3. Become defensive and attempt to discredit the results.
4. Develop excuses for why a particular outcome metric was high.
5. Question the accuracy of the data source.
6. Become stuck in the minutiae of details and fail to see the big picture.
7. State that administrative data isn't reflective of clinical practice.

Overcoming these critiques is an obstacle, but valid and reliable results along with a confident and effective graphical representation redirect the focus from discounting results towards driving improvement. The best offense is a great defense. Knowing the nuances of the methodology and the statistics of what is displayed reinforces credibility.

In today's busy environment, the advancement of technology means access to a massive amount of data, leading to information overload. Healthcare professionals are inundated with data and may make decisions with a limited understanding of the statistics and methodology behind the results, leading to a snowball effect of limited improvement. Does the snowball start with the wrong question about the right problem or the wrong interpretation of the right statistics? This creates an atmosphere where time is limited to interpret thousands of metrics requiring attention that impact organizational goals, financial and/or performance incentives, and individual goals. The critiques above stem from a lack of understanding of the data or biased hunches, beliefs, or thoughts based on experience, which detracts from the story being told by the visual display. This leads to individuals becoming defensive and asking the wrong question. This wrong question may ultimately result in an ineffective use of time, money, and resources. Developing an approach to systematically evaluate data effectively moves the discussion from being reactive to becoming proactive. The real question is how to methodologically encourage healthcare professionals to critically evaluate data and develop the right analytic question. This is easier said than done, but with the proper tools and mindset it can be accomplished.

Asking the right analytic question begins with having a process; searching for the appropriate question and future improvement initiatives is a journey with many forks and obstacles in the road. While it is important to know the destination, focusing only on the outcome and not the processes leading to the desired outcome will not fix the problem. Performance improvement and research is a journey, not a destination. Utilizing a methodological approach for critically thinking about what questions to ask begins with a proper plan, so STOP and think prior to asking questions.

- S: SMART goal – determining what question to ask begins with understanding the goal of where to improve.
- T: Think critically – leverage the skills learned about analyzing metrics and testing your creativity by understanding the data that's presented.
- O: Operationalization of your metrics – think from a methodological perspective about how to DEFINE variables (i.e., construct validity) to better understand how metrics are measured.
- P: Purpose – proper planning prevents poor performance. This purpose could be to develop a behavioral intervention or having a plan to accomplish your goal.

The most important aspect of the STOP tool is to have a plan for what is being accomplished. Every fork in the journey towards improvement presents an opportunity to STOP and think about where you want to go. Don't ever lose sight of the 50,000-foot view by getting stuck in the weeds. Likewise, don't get stuck in the 50,000-foot view trying to accomplish something that won't work. Think back to the purpose of what you want to accomplish. The STOP tool is versatile and can be utilized before the FACTS to create a sense of purpose and/or after focusing on the FACTS to strategize for the future. The end result is either developing a plan on where to focus improvement efforts or determining the future next steps. Moving beyond the FACTS presented and asking critical questions is the start of the process to internalize the story and formulate questions that move thinking to the next level. A methodological approach to search for the right analytic question is challenging, but the STOP tool is designed to force continual critical thinking.

When taking into consideration all the available healthcare data, the primary focus is on designing interventions to improve patient outcomes or some may argue to focus on government initiatives aimed at financial/performance incentives. Healthcare organizations exist due to patients, but without healthcare professionals, there would be no one to take care of these patients. Patients generate the majority of data that results in trending outcomes but ignoring input from healthcare professionals delivering the care is a mistake. Healthcare professionals have a powerful voice and a unique perspective on a variety of issues within the healthcare delivery process that is valuable to incorporate into interventions aimed to improve care. The Agency for Healthcare Research and Quality's (AHRQ) mission is devoted to evidence-based practice to ensure healthcare is "safer, higher quality, more accessible, equitable, and affordable, and to work within the U.S. Department of Health and Human Services" (www.ahrq.gov/cpi/about/index. html?).

AHRQ works with healthcare professionals and policymakers to ensure the necessary knowledge and data are used to make decisions. Their work has generated significant tools that have made healthcare safer through research and materials used to teach and train healthcare organizations and professionals. They are a believer in implementing **translational research** into practice, a concept known as **evidence-based practice**. AHRQ is credited with many tools, such as TeamSTEPPS, Healthcare Cost and Utilization Project (HCUP), EvidenceNOW, Comprehensive Unit-based Safety Program (CUSP), and the Consumer Assessment of Healthcare Providers and Systems (CAHPS). AHRQ continues to determine effective tools to address healthcare challenges in the future. One particular tool developed in 2004 by AHRQ was the patient safety survey that is administered to healthcare providers (i.e., hospitals, medical offices, nursing homes, community pharmacies, and ambulatory surgery centers) to assess the culture of safety. This survey provides an opportunity for healthcare professionals to voice concerns regarding patient safety. The perspective of these healthcare providers delivers the missing component on how to incorporate healthcare professionals' viewpoints into interventions driven to improve patient outcomes.

Why Focus on Patient Safety?

Obtaining multiple perspectives is an effective approach to driving improvement. Focusing on only administrative or EMR data will provide the perspective of the patient and outcomes related to that person. Healthcare data is multifaceted in that patients are not the only people to generate data. Healthcare professionals have a different perspective from that of patients and gathering their input is equally valuable.

The relationship between patient safety, patient outcomes, and patient experience has been readily studied, demonstrating an important link between a patient safety culture and patient outcomes (DiCuccio, 2015; Mardon, Khanna, Sorra, Dyer, & Famolaro, 2010; Weaver, Lubomski, Wilson, Pfoh, Martinez, & Dy, 2013). Researchers have found evidence of the relationship between patient safety culture, patient outcomes at the hospital, and the nursing staff's level of analysis (DiCuccio, 2015). Further research is mixed regarding the improvement in patient safety and patient outcomes (Weaver et al., 2013). However, Weaver et al. (2013) suggest that interventions improve patient safety and reduce patient harm and/or adverse events (Mardon et al., 2010).

Regardless of individual perceptions about the advantages/disadvantages of a culture of safety, the safety and quality of health care continue to be a focus as the relationship between patient harm and culture of safety is explored (Vogus, Sutcliffe, & Weick, 2010). AHRQ continues to promote relationships between patient safety and outcomes in order to drive improvement. The only challenge is how to operationalize and measure a culture of patient safety. AHRQ has developed a variety of surveys to assess metrics related to patient safety in various healthcare organizations.

One common critique of any survey design is the accuracy to which the measured domains are valid and reliable. No survey or measurement instrument will be 100% accurate, so some degree of error associated with the measurements is common and should not detract from the story of the results. Blegen, Gearhart, O'Brien, Sehgal, and Alldredge (2009) and Sorra and Dyer (2010) conducted psychometric analyses to assess the validity and reliability of the AHRQ patient safety survey and found all domains within the AHRQ survey, with the exception of the staffing subscale, to be valid and reliable measures of assessing patient safety culture.

Survey Methodology

Designing and administering surveys is common within many industries. Despite the potential measurement issues and response rates, there are methodological approaches to ensure a valid and reliable survey. Many of the concepts from within the patient experience chapter apply to this one with two additional important factors: sample responding and survey items.

Sample Responding

Having a voice in directing future initiatives is powerful. Ensuring those voices are heard is a separate issue. The main differentiation between patient experience and the safety survey is that patients respond to patient experience surveys and employees respond to the patient safety survey. The challenges faced when conducting surveys with patients versus employees are slightly different. Despite the safety survey being anonymous, employees may feel their individual responses are tracked and may not respond to the survey for fear of being identified or responding to the survey with desirable behaviors. Overcoming this obstacle begins with communicating and reinforcing that results are anonymous and are used to develop new interventions. Without a voice, changes cannot occur. Individuals completing surveys have a desire to express their views and experiences as well as to see results from their responses. Knowing they have a voice and seeing action being taken may result in improving response rates in future surveys.

One common question is the topic of response rate and how to improve it. A detriment to future survey response rates is not sharing results with those who have completed it. While a response rate is critical to ensure the validity of the results, average survey response rates range between 20% and 30% (Cook, Heath, & Thompson, 2000; Kaplowitz, Hadlock, & Levine, 2004). There is no guarantee for increasing response rates, but there are techniques to improve them. Dillman (2007) suggests four points of contact to maximize response rates: pre-survey letter, survey being sent, additional communication, then a follow-up reminder/thank you. The contact type could be a postcard, flyer posted in public view, electronic communications (i.e., email or a screen saver), etc. Multiple points of contact, which include follow-up reminders, have been shown to improve response rates (Cook et al., 2000) and reduce non-response bias (Barclay, Todd, Finlay, Grande, & Wyatt, 2002), which enhances the external validity of the results.

Keep in mind the AHRQ safety survey is administered to the entire population or a sample of the population based on utilizing a systematic or simple random sampling technique. When sampling employees for participation in the patient safety survey, it's important to ensure that an appropriate sample size is collected. AHRQ provides recommendations for a minimum sample size. Regardless of a sample being selected or surveying the entire population, not everyone will respond. Therefore, the results are based on the sample from the population that responded. To ensure the sample of responses is externally valid, compare the sample demographics to the population demographics. A sample representative of the population has higher external validity than a sample not representative of the population. The concern is the employees who did not respond. This is an issue of non-response bias, where the beliefs of employees not completing the survey differ from those of the employees who do respond. Following the methodology for multiple point of contact can improve response rates and reduce issues of non-response bias (Armstrong & Overton, 1977; Barclay et al., 2002; Cook et al., 2000).

Survey Items

The way in which survey questions or items are written has the ability to influence responses to a survey. It's imperative that items are written appropriately to maximize the results. Response scales (Mazaheri & Theuns, 2009; Russell & Carroll, 1999) and survey item construction have been shown to impact survey responses (Barnette, 2000; Horan, DiStefano, & Motl, 2003; Vautier, Callahan, Moncany, & Sztulman, 2004; Vautier & Pohl, 2009). Survey item construction is often leveraged to enhance the validity of the results and reduce survey **rating errors**. When individuals respond to a survey, possible rating errors are: leniency, halo, and central tendency errors.

- Leniency – ratings that are higher or lower than actual performance
- Halo – providing similar ratings across various measures of performance
- Central tendency – ratings consistently using the middle of the response scale.

There are a couple of ways to deal with rating errors. The first would be to utilize statistical methods to assess the impact of rating errors. An indication of leniency error is the presence of average ratings that are above the middle of the rating scale. A method to determine if halo rating errors exist is to examine the correlations between different metrics and standard deviations. If the result is a high correlation or small standard deviation, then it's plausible that halo rating errors exist. A means of assessing central tendency rating errors involves examining the distribution of the ratings where values would congregate towards the center or having a small standard deviation (Lutsky, Risucci, & Tortolani, 1993).

One way to combat rating errors is through negatively worded items or **reverse-scored items**. An example is when, instead of saying "there are patient safety problems," the question is negatively worded to say "there are no patient safety problems." The AHRQ patient safety survey utilizes this technique as a mechanism to ensure individuals carefully read each survey item. Inconsistent responses are eliminated due to the occurrence of a rating error. While the ultimate goal is to ensure the validity of survey responses and elicit honest feedback, reducing any rating error is advantageous to protect the integrity of the results. The caveat to negatively worded items is they add to the cognitive burden of the individual responding to the survey by forcing them to think about each item. While this may be considered a good thing, negatively worded questions pose a potential problem of how individuals may interpret the question, which results in providing an answer that may not reflect how they feel. Consider the question mentioned above of "there are patient safety problems" and the reverse-scored item of "there are no patient safety problems." In this case answering in the negative is preferred as you would want no safety problems. Understanding whether or not a "no" is considered a negative or positive response is desirable may increase the cognitive burden on the survey taker.

In conclusion, there are three potential issues to consider with surveys: (1) improving response rates; (2) sample of responses similar to the population or responses are similar to non-responses; and (3) influence of how survey item is written (i.e., reverse-scored items) to eliminate rating errors. All three of these issues are important to consider when administering any type of survey. Not all of this is avoidable and any potential issue with a survey could compromise the validity of the results. Keep in mind that any survey or metric involved with measuring human behavior is likely to have a degree of error associated with the actual measurement. Despite this potential error, many organizations utilize surveys to effectively drive change through accountability and sharing results in a timely manner.

AHRQ Hospital Survey Methodology

AHRQ has various surveys available for measuring patient safety, but the focus for this chapter is the hospital survey. Refer to the AHRQ website (www.ahrq. gov/) for further information regarding the other patient safety surveys, which are medical office, nursing home, community pharmacy, and ambulatory surgery center. When analyzing the AHRQ hospital patient safety survey, reflect on the methodology AHRQ recommends to collect data. The patient safety survey is a self-administered survey given to all employees with the recommendation of administration every 18 months. The hospital survey consists of 42 questions plus demographic questions that comprise a total of 12 domains. The individual questions are rated on a 5-point Likert-type scale from strongly disagree to strongly agree, with negatively worded questions to be reverse-scored. Responses are aggregated into percentages with benchmarks available on a variety of demographic questions and drill downs to department and position, if eligible. The one stipulation is that drill downs on questions can only be done with 10 or more responses for a given demographic. The 12 hospital survey domains are as follows:

1. Teamwork within units
2. Supervisor/manager expectations and actions promoting patient safety
3. Organizational learning – continuous improvement
4. Management support for patient safety
5. Overall perceptions of patient safety
6. Feedback and communication about error
7. Communication openness
8. Frequency of events reported
9. Teamwork across units
10. Staffing
11. Handoffs and transitions
12. Non-punitive response to errors.

Continuing with a methodological approach, step back before analyzing the results by focusing on how the domains are defined from a construct validity perspective. The DEFINE tool is effective for understanding how metrics are analyzed, but utilize it for providing a methodological framework to operationalize a measure or domain. Using the DEFINE tool for the hospital communication openness domain reveals the following:

- Denominator – all employees responding to the survey
- Exclusion criteria – any employee not in a hospital setting or volunteers
- Factor – to be determined based on reviewing metrics within AHRQ. Responses on a Likert-type scale are analyzed as averages/means or converted to percentages
- Inclusion criteria – any full-time, part-time, or per diem employees
- Numerator – survey responses based on the average or potential top/bottom responses
- Evaluate – in reviewing AHRQ, there are three items measuring this domain with one negatively worded item. Review the content of the items to understand how it is measured.

Take the time to review what questions are used to assess a given domain. This is important, because when developing interventions aimed at improving domains, the intervention must be related to the items being assessed. It is not possible to improve a domain when the intervention does not address the items being measured. Continuing with the communication openness domain, there are three items with one negatively worded one.

1. Staff will freely speak up if they see something that may negatively affect patient care.
2. Staff feel free to question the decisions or actions of those with more authority.
3. Staff are afraid to ask questions when something does not seem right (negatively worded).

When developing an intervention aimed at improving communication openness, notice the survey defines this domain as speaking up when patient care is in jeopardy, feeling free to question decisions or actions of authority, and fear of asking questions when something isn't right. An intervention created that encourages a flow of communication may not specifically address the questions being measured, which could result in no improvement on future administrations.

While the DEFINE tool may have some gaps in the initial exploration process, it forces thinking to structure concepts into the format of a metric. Once the discussion moves beyond the operationalization of the domain, the DEFINE tool provides structure to develop the metric. Utilizing the communication openness domain, a metric is defined as follows:

- Denominator – total number of responses for the communication openness domain
- Exclusion criteria – incomplete surveys having less than half the questions answered or the same response for all questions (i.e., rating errors)
- Factor – rate multiplied by 100
- Inclusion criteria – full-time, part-time, and per diem employees
- Numerator – total positive responses, defined as the top two responses for positively worded items and the bottom two responses for negatively worded items
- Evaluate – communication openness is a rate based on positive perceptions of questions containing the top two responses for respective questions multiplied by 100. All responses are included except for incomplete survey responses (missing or rating errors). There were three questions, with one being negatively worded. Questions indicate this domain is related to speaking up/questioning authority or patient care.

The presentation of results is critical for two interrelated reasons: (1) potential impact on future responses and response rates to the same survey; and (2) leveraging results to drive change and take action. Individuals appreciate knowing action is taken from surveys they opted to voluntarily complete. When there is an appearance of no action from results, the tendency to complete future surveys may decline. This creates the need to ensure results from surveys are analyzed appropriately and presented back to the individuals who took the time to complete them with demonstrated interventions aimed at improving issues employees identified.

The complicated aspect of analyzing surveys to drive change is based on the volume of available data and external validity of the results from the sample to the population. For instance, aggregating results from 12 domains and 42 questions on the AHRQ patient safety survey is complicated. There are many ways to analyze the data, but creatively presenting results that tells a story and generates more questions than answers is challenging. Jumping into the results without taking a step back to think about the bigger picture leads to information overload due to ineffectively thinking about how to effectively present the results.

A methodological approach to information gathering prior to analyzing results ensures all available information is utilized prior to creating a graphical representation. In other words, it's critical to know the data and what is available. Presenting results of an organization's response to the survey is effective, but adding comparative benchmarks enhances the context of the story to provide comparisons to other organizations. AHRQ utilizes a comparative database with benchmarks by domain for a variety of demographics, such as regions within the United States, bed size, teaching status, etc. There is value for not only analyzing internal performance, but also stepping outside the organization to compare performance metrics to externally similar organizations across domains. Incorporating multiple viewpoints both internally and externally aids in the search for the critical questions to ask. You can't be number 1 if you don't know how number 1 is doing.

Prior to analyzing the results, review the methodological requirements for sharing results so anonymity is protected. AHRQ provides two points to consider: (1) there must be more than 10 responses for a department/position to display survey item level results; and (2) interpretation for improvement is based on two predefined categories, which are that values of less than 50% indicates an opportunity for improvement and greater than 75% as an area of strength. Utilizing comparative benchmarks becomes critical as some national benchmarks in the nationwide comparative report score below 50% in certain domains.

When presenting the results, a variety of options are available to display data in meaningful ways. Any piece of information included within a survey is valuable, so don't forget to leverage the analysis of demographic questions and national benchmarks to maximize multiple viewpoints when storytelling with data. Additionally, take advantage of the power of statistics if the organization has the raw data. The statistical analysis conducted when raw data is available is robust and powerful compared to only having descriptive data. Raw data allows the opportunity to analyze results at a high level and drill down to departments/positions and calculate statistics, such as means, standard deviation, confidence intervals, regression techniques, p values, or statistical significance to enhance the story. Just be mindful that AHRQ recommends more than 10 responses for a department/position to protect the anonymity of the results.

Results

The wealth of information available for the AHRQ patient safety survey is overwhelming to analyze considering there are 12 domains and 42 questions.

Nurturing Target Audiences

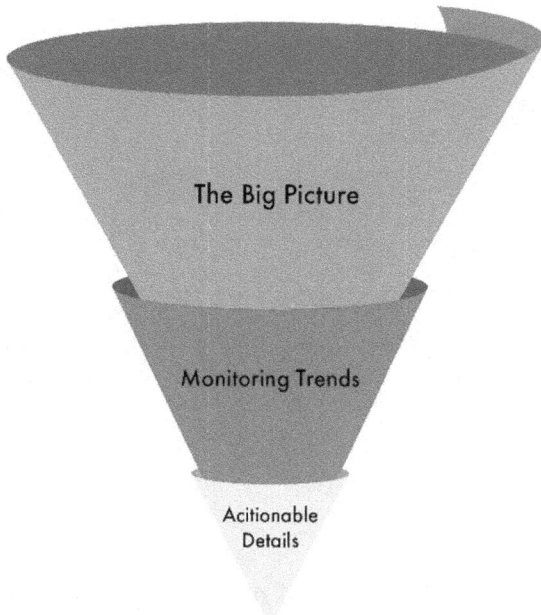

Figure 6.1 Funnel-down approach.

Jumping into the details of the results is not an effective methodological approach to tell the story. Take a step back and start at a higher level and then drill down to the details of the results. This approach is referred to as the funnel-down approach to presenting results (Figure 6.1).

In utilizing this funnel-down approach, the presentation of the results begins with an overview of the entire survey. Step back and think big picture! If an organization is administering the hospital patient safety survey to multiple hospitals, then focusing on the high-level results (i.e., overall domains) across hospitals within the organization would be at the top of the funnel. This sets the stage of the story by allowing leaders to view a snapshot of the entire organization to determine opportunities for improvement and areas of strength. An example of this high-level analysis is provided in Figure 6.2.

Graphical representations of data make it easy to jump to conclusions and make decisions without a systematic methodological approach to critical thinking. There are many stories using statistics at face value, but step back and focus on the FACTS.

- Formulas – rate is calculated as a positive perception of the questions within the domain.

3:33/1

HEALTH ORGANIZATION	COMMUNICATION OPENNESS	FEEDBACK AND COMMUNICATION ABOUT ERROR	FREQUENCY OF EVENTS REPORTED	HOSPITAL HANDOFFS & TRANSITIONS	HOSPITAL MANAGEMENT SUPPORT FOR PATIENT SAFETY	NONPUNITIVE RESPONSE TO ERROR	ORGANIZATIONAL LEARNING-CONTINUOUS IMPROVEMENT	OVERALL PERCEPTIONS OF SAFETY	STAFFING	SUPERVISOR/MANAGER EXPECTATIONS & ACTIONS PROMOTING PATIENT SAFETY	TEAMWORK ACROSS HOSPITAL UNITS	TEAMWORK WITHIN UNITS
HOSPITAL A	63.9	72.2	72.6	62.7	80.0	45.8	75.7	68.6	42.9	77.9	72.4	80.6
HOSPITAL B	69.4	77.6	74.5	51.2	74.6	47.1	77.7	71.7	55.7	79.8	64.6	80.1
HOSPITAL C	69.7	76.1	78.0	45.4	76.2	43.8	79.1	70.5	52.2	76.5	63.2	82.2
HOSPITAL D	65.8	74.7	73.7	48.2	71.9	41.8	76.0	63.3	51.8	75.5	59.0	77.7
HOSPITAL E	69.7	78.1	75.1	59.1	79.4	50.8	78.6	78.0	66.9	79.6	69.8	81.5
OVERALL TOTAL	65.3	74.6	73.6	48.9	73.4	42.3	76.7	66.8	50.7	75.4	61.1	79.9

▨ Area of Strength

▨ Potential for Improvement

✓ Better than or Equal to National Average

Figure 6.2 Big picture funnel.

- Analyze patterns/trends – initial pattern and trend appear to demonstrate an opportunity for non-punitive response to errors, hospital handoffs and transitions, and an area of strength for teamwork within units and organizational learning – continuous improvement.
- Consider rules/guidelines – AHRQ rules indicate < 50% as an opportunity for improvement and > 75% as an area of strength.
- Think methodologically – rules are arbitrary cutoffs, so combining rules with national benchmarks aid in the interpretation. Focus on individual hospital domain scores in relation to national benchmarks.
- Statistics – average rates for the hospital, organization, and comparisons to national benchmarks

This snapshot of a health organization can stimulate significant conversations, but the path towards improvement is hidden within the data. With only one perspective of the organization's data, it's easy to jump to conclusions and state the organization has an opportunity for improvement with non-punitive response to error and an area of strength for teamwork within units. When bringing into perspective the comparative benchmarks, a slightly different story emerges. Notice that, for non-punitive response to error, Hospital A has a score of 45.8% and is higher than the national rate. This indicates that, while it is an opportunity for improvement, the entire AHRQ comparative database also scores as an area of opportunity. With respect to teamwork within units, most hospitals score above 75%, which indicates an area of strength. However, notice that very few hospitals are above the national average. There are two conclusions: (1) an opportunity for improvement does not always indicate this domain is a primary focus when the national benchmarks indicate the domain, as a whole, is an opportunity for improvement; and (2) an area of strength still presents opportunities for improvement when compared to national benchmarks.

Analytics, when presented effectively, generate more questions than answers. The purpose of the analysis is to promote critical thinking to guide the next phase of the results. After viewing the big picture from the top of the funnel, drill down to the overall hospital performance on the entire survey with benchmark comparisons. The high-level analysis provides an overall picture of each domain individually. Hospitals should be concerned with the overall domain score, but also the response rate and demographics of the sample responses. By understanding the response rate and sample that responded, the external validity of the results from the current sample is established through comparing sample characteristics to the entire hospital population. This analysis is helpful to debunk attempts at criticizing the data as not being representative of the population.

Determining the type of graphical representation depends on the amount of data that was collected at various points in time. As mentioned before, AHRQ recommends administering the survey every 18 months, so multiple administrations allow the ability to create run or control charts; assuming more than 18 data points are available for a control chart. Trended data allows the examination of patterns/trends over the course of time to determine/monitor improvement efforts. However, run/control charts may not always be the answer. Having the raw data and utilizing a methodological approach with a little creativity may yield a different mode of presentation. Perhaps the decision is to examine variability in responses, because any type of response to the survey is valuable. Moving down from the top of the funnel indicates the analytics are narrow in scope, so in this case the analytics move from the health organization/hospital level for all domains down towards the individual domains. Figure 6.3 provides a bar chart analyzing the communication openness domain with individual responses to each of the three questions. Even with limited statistics being presented, it's critical to continue to focus on the FACTS.

- Formulas – rates calculated by the percent agreement. The 5-point Likert-type scale is condensed to three responses where responses of 1 and 2 are combined and responses 4 and 5 are combined to create the top 2 and bottom 2 box.
- Analyze patterns/trends – question 1 is higher than the national rate. Question 2 provides significant opportunity for improvement. Question 3 provides variable responses, but mostly positive (keep in mind this is reverse-scored, so %never/rarely is positive).
- Consider rules/guidelines – compare individual items to the national rate for communication openness.
- Think methodologically – focus on individual items and notice that one item is reverse-scored, so the 60% would be ideal, whereas the 80% and 55% of the other two items are ideal. Examine each item to know what the question is assessing.
- Statistics – percentages.

3:33/2

COMMUNICATION OPENNESS (N=1,363)

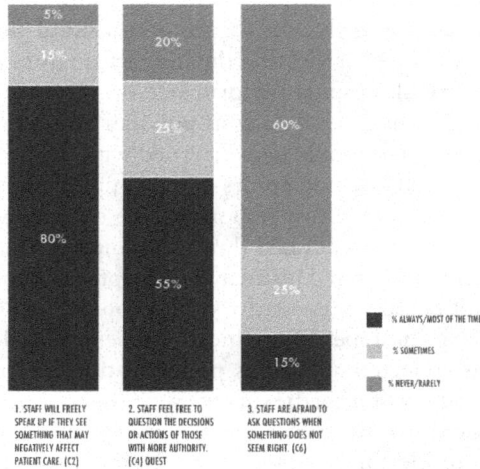

Figure 6.3 Middle of the funnel hospital level.

The variability in average rates provides further insight on where to focus. Utilizing the national rate as a benchmark allows a comparison of the individual items to drive improvement. Assume that the national rate for communication openness is 63%. This indicates that questions 2 (55%) and 3 (60%) (recall question 3 is reverse-scored, so %never/rarely is more desirable) provide an opportunity for improvement as they are both below the 63%. When examining the content of the question, the theme is concerned with questioning those in authority and being afraid to ask questions when something is not right.

At this point the funnel-down approach yields an overall domain score compared to national rates and other hospitals and the hospital analysis provides a more detailed look at responses to questions within the domain. Knowing the methodology of the survey and having the raw data means there are further analyses available. Assuming more than 10 responses, the funnel-down approach narrows from the domain level to the department or position level. Comparing responses at the domain or individual survey item level across departments to the benchmarked data further enhances the story. Refer to Figure 6.4 for responses by department and Table 6.1 for department level responses to individual survey items. The FACTS of the story, which includes formulas and statistics, have not changed, so focus on where to ACT.

• Analyze patterns/trends – there is a wide gap between the top department, pediatrics (81.0%), and the lowest department, emergency department (56.1%).

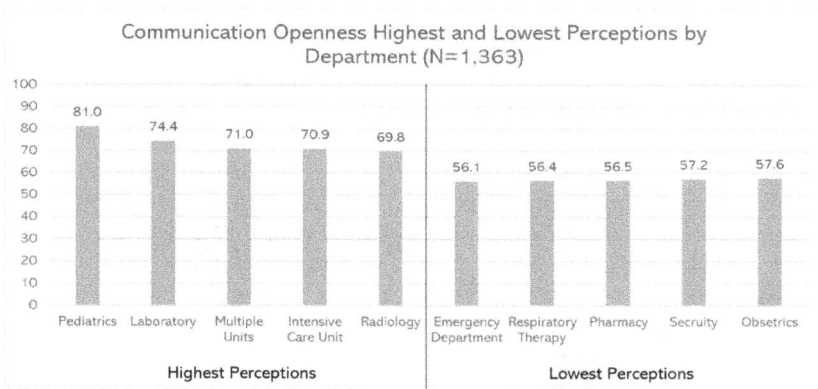

Communication Openness Highest and Lowest Perceptions by Department (N=1,363)

Figure 6.4 Bottom of funnel graphical representation of individual departments (high and low performers) on communication openness domain.

Table 6.1 Department performance by question

Questions	Department	Score (%)	n
Communication openness domain	Intensive care unit	70.9	244
	Obstetrics	57.6	201
	Pediatrics	81.0	57
	Emergency department	56.1	131
1. Staff will freely speak up if they see something that may negatively affect patient care (C2)	Intensive care unit	84.8	244
	Obstetrics	72.1	201
	Pediatrics	86.0	57
	Emergency department	56.9	130
2. Staff feel free to question the decisions or actions of those with more authority (C4)	Intensive care unit	61.1	244
	Obstetrics	51.2	201
	Pediatrics	66.7	57
	Emergency department	68.4	131
3. Staff are afraid to ask questions when something does not seem right (C6)	Intensive care unit	64.2	243
	Obstetrics	53.0	200
	Pediatrics	80.7	57
	Emergency department	42.7	131

- Consider rules/guidelines – the national domain rate (assume 63%) is a combination of three items. Overall, the intensive care unit and pediatrics are above the national rate and an area of strength. Obstetrics and emergency department are below the national rate, but don't meet the 50% opportunity for improvement. Examining department individual item performances shows even top-performing departments have opportunities for improvement and low-performing departments have areas of strength.

- Think methodologically – using the 75% and 50% cutoffs as areas of strength or opportunities for improvement is one approach. Using the comparative database for national benchmarks provides added performance opportunities. Variability in scores indicates multiple opportunities for process improvement.

Focusing on the overall domain score and not drilling down paints a different picture of where to focus improvement efforts. While the pediatrics department scored high on communication openness, the FACTS identify a common theme of issues questioning actions of authority (the emergency department scored the highest on that item, 68.4%). There are opportunities for sharing information across departments that are lost when focusing on the higher-level results. This is the benefit of utilizing a methodological funnel-down approach for analytics when you have access to raw data.

You have two options to choose from when analyzing data: (1) utilize AHRQ guidelines for area of strength (scores > 75%) or opportunities for improvement (scores < 50%); or (2) take into consideration comparisons to the national rates as provided in AHRQ's comparative database. Aiming for above the national rate is an achievement, but this benchmark is a moving target. Likewise, focusing on the opportunity for improvement (scores < 50%) could have you improving a metric (non-punitive response to error) when the entire country is below 50%. Determining where to focus begins with a plan. All analytics answer some questions, but likely there are more questions than answers. As a result, STOP and think about a plan for improvement.

- SMART goal – develop an intervention to improve confidence with "question actions of others with more authority" by 10% during the next survey administration.
- Think critically – best practice initiatives come from multiple departments. Leverage statistical knowledge to conduct focus groups with departments to share best practices.
- Operationalize your metrics – define what employees mean when interpreting decisions or actions and who they consider as having more authority, especially if negatively worded questions exist.
- Purpose – conduct a focus group to operationalize metrics and learn from various departments to let them know you're listening and want to improve.

A methodological funnel-down approach to analyzing statistics eliminates biases and assumptions. Reacting to results at face value without thinking creates ineffective improvement efforts. Limited time/resources to analyze data and relying on overall system/hospital level results may end up with missed opportunities. As can be seen from this analysis, the initial focus of where to improve may change as more information (i.e., national benchmarks, department/position level, and/or specific item results) becomes known or leveraged. Taking action based on department level results only would exclude pediatrics from being analyzed as this was the highest-performing department. Focusing on individual survey items revealed the emergency department was outperforming pediatrics on one item, which indicates that, regardless of performance, there is some lesson to be learned from high- and low-performers.

Discussion

Data has a significant amount of power for guiding the story and driving future questions when an organization has the raw data. A methodological funnel-down approach to analyzing statistics generates more questions than answers, but ensures all analyses are objectively evaluated by removing assumptions, hunches, and beliefs. Ponder the following thoughts:

1. How do you overcome the hesitation of self-identification? Drilling down to department/position results of individual survey items is powerful for guiding the development of behavioral interventions.
2. It is important to step back and not jump to conclusions from the results taken at face value and methodologically approach the survey design.
3. An analysis of data should generate more questions than answers to further direct improvement efforts.

The first issue to consider is overcoming the challenge of being able to encourage respondents to self-identify. This is easier said than done. How does someone convince another individual that results are anonymous and confidential, so they cannot be identified? Fear of identification could result in responses that lead to socially desirable answers (Wildman, 1977) or questions about whether or not employees are telling the truth (Hyman, 1944). Would employees respond favorably or truthfully if there is a potential that their responses are not confidential and anonymous? Ong and Weiss (2000) found the responses from surveys that were deemed anonymous resulted in a greater percentage of individuals acknowledging a behavior compared to responses that were deemed confidential. The only self-identification on the survey is a department/unit and position. If possible, analyzing this data at the individual position level leads to more information than aggregating at a system/hospital level where some knowledge can be lost. AHRQ rules require 10 or more responses, so results for smaller areas and positions cannot be statistically analyzed without self-identification.

The second issue of having a methodological approach to survey design will aid in the interpretation of the results. Surveys are complex self-report instruments designed to capture information from an individual to better understand the phenomenon of interest. Every construct defined within a survey carries its own connotation. Not everyone may define a metric exactly the same way. New constructs are created regularly and researchers defend constructs due to the social implications they carry (Picardi & Masick, 2013). Knowing how each domain on the AHRQ patient safety survey is defined ensures a clear understanding of how to improve this measure. This is the difference between *thinking* and *knowing* what to do. Remember the communication openness domain and the three items used to measure it? The introduction of a reverse-scored item on a survey or the way questions are phrased could influence how someone may define each individual item. Think about your response to the question of "rate your overall level of satisfaction/dissatisfaction with your total compensation." Does the term total compensation refer to your salary or your salary plus any bonus, paid time off, health benefits, work/life balance benefits, tuition assistance, work from home, flexible work schedules, etc?

The third issue is that when results are analyzed and presented in an effective way, a clear story emerges, leading to the formulation of new questions or needing further information to drive change. This is important because, when analyzing data, the questions asked are as important as the results of the analysis. Think about the example of data presented in the health organization (Figure 6.2) and hospital domain graph (Figure 6.3) compared to the results found when analyzing individual department level item scores (Figure 6.4 and Table 6.1). Did the analytics presented in both scenarios lead to the same question or drive the same improvement efforts?

Being able to analyze the statistical information is beneficial, but knowing where to go and how to drill down is equally important. Surveys provide one aspect of what is happening. An additional way of being able to drill down to the root cause of a problem is to conduct focus groups. You can only hypothesize what is happening within a department. If you're not there 24 hours a day 7 days a week, then you really don't know what's happening. Why not conduct a focus group in the department or area of interest to better understand what is happening? This is also an effective way of sharing the survey results. There is always something to be learned when gathering additional information, so why not focus on high- and low-domain scores? There is a lot to learn from high-performing departments as well. One may argue that it is not possible to compare results across departments. While this may be true in aspects of care delivery, staffing models, and patient acuity, there are likely behavioral-based competencies that transcend these differences. Breaking these components/behaviors into processes and outcomes is possible and may be beneficial for sharing best practice.

The main overarching theme of this chapter was that asking questions is as critical as analyzing results. The results are only one piece of the puzzle. The STOP tool is one technique to search for the critical question to ask in order to improve or change behavior. Aim the questions at understanding the process and gathering additional information to assist with setting goals or driving change. When considering a change in process to improve outcomes, it's beneficial to create a process map to better understand how the intervention impacts sustainable change. Keep in mind that you can't change what you don't measure and you can't act on what you don't ask. Driving any type of change towards improving behavior will not be successful without a proper plan. If you took the time to methodologically approach and analyze statistics, then don't skip the plan. Take the time to STOP and formulate a plan to hit those moving targets.

Discussion Questions

- Compare and contrast your views on whether statistics provide answers or generate more questions than answers.

- What types of techniques do you do to be proactive with future initiatives as opposed to reacting to situations as they arise?
- Other than the list of criticisms of the validity of the data, are there any other criticisms you have heard?
- Have you ever made improvement decisions without fully understanding the statistics or methodology? What was the end result?
- Is it possible to take results at face value and effectively initiate change?
- How does a combination of healthcare patient data combined with healthcare professional data help to drive improvements in patient outcomes?
- Does the idea of non-response bias, where there may be a difference between those who respond to the survey versus those that don't, concern you with making improvement decisions? Why or why not?
- What methods have you used to improve response rates or ensure the sample is representative of the population when administering a survey?
- What type of interventions have you implemented utilizing the safety survey or any other survey to drive change? Was it successful? Did future administrations of that survey demonstrate improvements?
- Making decisions on where to focus improvement efforts is a challenge. Focusing on opportunities for improvement is valuable, but areas of strength may also be important. What is your decision-making process for driving change?

7   Past, Present, and Future

The Evolution of Initiatives

"There are always three stories: what happened, what is happening, what will happen."

Introduction

The evolution of change within healthcare creates the need to better understand the past, present, and where the future may go. As we know, the best predictor of future behavior is past performance (Wernimont & Campbell, 1968). The way care is being delivered today may not be the same in the future, but understanding what happened in the past can be an indicator as to what may happen in the future. There is no doubt that healthcare delivery is transforming, whether this change is focusing on the entire continuum of care, quality tied to performance, transition from inpatient services to outpatient services, etc. Regardless of the future direction, focusing on the hospital's four walls is no longer effective for maintaining a competitive edge. Organizations not only provide a service but are assessed on how well they manage patient care outcomes. Continued innovation and stretching our ability beyond what is imaginable lead to innovation. Be the innovator disruptors in healthcare to drive future improvement. It's not possible to change what happened in the past; it may be hard to change the present, but the future hasn't yet been written.

Government initiatives are changing the way hospitals deliver care, such as focusing on bundled payments to manage care outside the hospital or pay for performance to reward hospitals for meeting performance-based goals. Many different types of initiatives exist that make it not possible to cover every initiative in detail. Additionally, the constant change that occurs within initiatives makes it challenging to stay on top of the requirements. To remain consistent with our approach to analyze data, the focus is on the methodological aspect to these various initiatives to methodologically analyze the past, present, and future. The following is a list of some government initiatives in healthcare today:

1.   Partnership for Patients
2.   Patient Protection and Affordable Care Act (ACA)
3.   Pay for Performance (P4P)

4. Value–Based Purchasing (VBP)
5. Hospital Readmissions Reduction Program (HRRP)
6. Hospital-Acquired Condition Reduction Program (HACRP)
7. Bundled Payments for Care Improvement (BPCI)
8. Core Measures and Bundled Treatment.

Partnership for Patients

Partnership for Patients is a Centers for Medicare/Medicaid Services (CMS) initiative (https://partnershipforpatients.cms.gov/) joined by over 8,000 hospitals,
national organizations, patient and consumer organizations, employees, and states
to focus on safe care or improved care transitions. A main goal of Partnership
for Patients is a 20% reduction in patient harm and 12% reduction in 30-day
readmissions. Reducing patient harm is evaluated through reductions in 11 areas
of patient harm: (1) adverse drug events; (2) central line-associated blood stream
infections (CLABSI); (3) catheter-associated urinary tract infections; (4) *Clostridium
difficile*; (5) injuries from falls and immobility; (6) pressure ulcers; (7) sepsis and septic
shock; (8) surgical site infections; (9) venous thromboembolism; (10) ventilator-
associated events; and (11) readmissions.

Patient Protection and Affordable Care Act

The Patient Protection and Affordable Care Act was shortened to the Affordable
Care Act or ACA and is also known as Obamacare (www.healthcare.gov/). The
ACA is a government healthcare reform law passed under President Barrack
Obama in 2010. This complex legislation consists of 974 pages (www.hhs.gov/
sites/default/files/ppacacon.pdf). The ACA is comprised of three goals: (1) affordable health insurance for more people based on subsidies by income; (2) expansion of Medicaid; and (3) support innovations to lower costs. A provision of ACA
resulted in the authorization of value-based payment programs, such as VBP,
HRRP, and HACRP. These programs are aimed at transitioning hospital-based
payment models to a pay-for-performance initiative towards improving quality,
reducing costs, and improving patient outcomes. Additionally, the ACA aimed to
lower the uninsured rate through an expansion of insurance coverage. With any
government initiative and the evolution of healthcare, the ACA may be altered in
the future.

Pay for Performance

P4P is an incentivized initiative that captures programs focused on improving
quality, efficiency, and value. This initiative is an aim to change healthcare incentive structure from a fee-for-service to pay-for-performance. The ACA contains
provisions designed towards payment models linked to quality and outcome. In
general, P4P or VBP is a broad term used to capture any program that results in
payments based on performance. P4P utilizes four categories: process measures,

outcome measures, patient experience, and structure. Process measures are chosen based on a demonstrated contribution to outcome measures. Patient experience measures aim to assess individual patients' perception of satisfaction and quality. Lastly, structure focuses on metrics corresponding to the actual facility, personnel, or equipment.

Value-Based Purchasing

CMS created VBP, also known as Hospital Value-Based Purchasing Program (HVBP), programs through the establishment of the ACA to change the way hospitals are paid. These programs are designed to pay hospitals receiving Medicare payments based on performance on a variety of metrics. Payments through this program are based on not only how well a hospital performs on metrics related to all hospitals, but how well hospitals perform in comparison to their prior baseline period for determining improvement. Metrics included within the VBP program are subject to change on a fiscal-year basis. Refer to the VBP website for the latest quality domains, weights, baseline/performance periods, scoring, and minimum eligibility associated with the program (www. qualitynet.org/inpatient/hvbp). From fiscal years (FY) 2019 through 2024, there are four domains: clinical care (outcomes and process), person and community engagement, safety, and efficiency and cost reduction (www.qualitynet. org). These four domains make up around 20 metrics, which may vary based on FY. In total, there are six clinical care metrics, eight person and community engagement metrics, PSI-90 (Patient Safety and Adverse Events Composite) and 5–6 hospital-acquired infection safety metrics, and Medicare spending per beneficiary for efficiency and cost reduction.

Hospital Readmissions Reduction Program

The HHRP was authorized as part of the ACA and results in a reduction in hospital payments due to excess readmissions with no financial incentives to earn more money. Hospital payments for Medicare are reduced based on a calculation of a readmission adjustment factor to account for excess readmissions. The goal of this program is to improve quality of care and care transitions that would incentivize hospitals towards reducing readmissions through increasing accountability of care. Readmission metrics included in the program are heart attack, heart failure, pneumonia, chronic obstructive pulmonary disease, hip/knee replacement, and coronary artery bypass graft surgery. Metrics included within this program are subject to change. Refer to the CMS website for current metrics www. cms.gov/Medicare/Medicare-Fee-for-Service-Payment/AcuteInpatientPPS/ Readmissions-Reduction-Program.html or https://qualitynet.org/inpatient/ hrrp/measures. New measures continue to be tested and developed, such as the excess days in acute care (EDAC) measure that educates clinicians on the delivery of care post discharge. The calculations are publicly available and hospitals are provided an opportunity to review and submit corrections to readmission rates prior to the results being publicly available.

Hospital–Acquired Condition Reduction Program

The HACRP is the final program under the ACA that authorizes CMS to reduce hospital payments based on performance calculated using percentiles. The goal of the program is to improve patient safety through a reduction in hospital-acquired conditions and adverse patent safety events. The HACRP is based on an overall HAC score comprised of six quality measures within two domains as of FY 2015–FY 2020. Domain 1 is the PSI-90 composite score and domain 2 is the following healthcare-associated infection (HAI) measures: CLABSI, catheter-associated urinary tract infection (CAUTI), colon and hysterectomy surgical site infection (SSI), methicillin-resistant *Staphylococcus aureus* (MRSA) bacteremia, *Clostridium difficile* infection (CDI). As with other initiatives, the HACRP is subject to change. Refer to the website (www.qualitynet.org) for up-to-date information. The HAC score is calculated by weighting domains 1 and 2, then converting scores into percentiles. The percentiles are divided into 10 equal deciles and reductions in payments are based on hospitals performing above the 75th percentile.

Bundled Payments for Care Improvement

A focus of the ACA has been to improve quality and affordability. Provisions within the ACA made it possible to shift Medicare payments to alternative payment models or population-based payments. The Department of Health and Human Services (HHS) tested and expanded payment models that improve quality and decrease cost through one overall payment designed to provide care over a specified period post hospitalization. The transition towards BPCI means hospitals are paid based on not only care received within the hospital, but for the entire continuum for up to 90 days following the hospitalization. To award payment based on episodes of care, CMS tested four broadly defined models in April 2013 and currently have 48 clinical episodes that participants are able to choose from. The CMS Innovation Center is continually testing and implementing new payment models, so check out their website (https://innovation.cms.gov/initiatives/bundled-payments).

Core Measures and Bundled Treatments

Core measures and bundled treatments are similar in context, but don't confuse bundled treatment with bundled payments. Core measures are treatment processes and standards of care for reducing complications, improving patient outcomes, and reliably delivering the right care to patients based on national standards. Bundled treatments are similar in scope but also utilize evidence-based practice for developing standards of treatment to improve patient outcomes. Over the years, CMS has implemented core measures to track compliance with certain medical conditions as a means to ensure all treatment processes are met. These core measures apply when delivering care to patients where certain protocols/processes are required for meeting the standard of care. The development of standards of care for treatment is a collaborative effort with healthcare professionals and other organizations. The end result for calculating statistics using core measures or bundled treatment uses an all-or-none compliance where all treatment processes in the bundle must be completed to be considered compliant.

For example, CMS developed a bundle treatment in collaboration with America's Health Insurance Plans (AHIP), National Quality Forum (NQF), and other national organizations to determine consensus on severe sepsis/septic shock. Consistent with the Surviving Sepsis Campaign guidelines, the CMS SEP-1 Early Management Bundle for Severe Sepsis/Septic Shock requires the following within 3 hours:

- Initial lactate level (lactate)
- Blood cultures drawn before antibiotics (blood cultures)
- Administration of antibiotics (antibiotics).

The remaining interventions must be completed within 6 hours: fluid resuscitation of 30 ml/kg crystalloid fluids (fluids), vassopressor administration, reassess volume status and tissue perfusion, and a repeat lactate measurement. Refer to the Joint Commission specification manual (www.jointcommission.org/specifications_manual_for_national_hospital_inpatient_quality_measures.aspx). Whether the initiative is referred to as core measures, bundled treatment, bundled compliance, or early management bundle, the outcome of completing all interventions to be considered compliant is the same.

Healthcare continues to change and evolve over time with new initiatives and buzz words emerging. Regardless of what initiatives/programs are available to healthcare organizations, new and innovative payment methods continue to be developed. Understanding the past and present is a good indicator for where the future is going. Metrics and their associated weights in the calculations may change, so review the most up-to-date information to know what is being measured and any metric impacting multiple initiatives. The above eight programs/initiatives are some of the many different models currently being used while others are continually developed to push the boundaries of delivering high-quality care. To hit those moving targets, stay one step ahead by regularly reviewing and knowing these initiatives to plan for the future.

A common question asked is, "what metric should we focus on?" This is not an easy answer, but a little research into the metrics of each initiatives may shed light on where to focus. Some metrics impact a performance scoring system, others have a financial penalty/incentive, and others have both performance and financial implications, so a low performance on a single metric can impact a variety of initiatives. For example, infection metrics appear in VBP, P4P, and HACRP that impact financial reimbursement and in the CMS Star Rating (Chapter 8) for ranking performance. As a result, lower performance on a single metric potentially impacts many aspects of a hospital's performance and financial incentives. A sample of relationships between the domains and a few of the programs are given in Table 7.1.

Methodology

One of the most effective ways to deal with change is to be proactive instead of reactive. Being proactive starts with understanding how you're being measured through various programs and determining what metrics to focus improvement efforts on. The patterns and trends from the past provide insight into where the future may go to help hit those moving targets. Programs/initiatives will change and new buzz words will emerge, so continually refer to the appropriate websites for the most up-to-date metrics and definitions.

The question posed earlier about "what metric should I focus on?" may lead to someone responding with, "all of them." It is an unrealistic approach to improve everything, so pick your battles wisely. All metrics have different impacts both financially and on performance with varying weights associated with how much they influence the outcome of that program/initiative. Knowing an organization's resources is not unlimited, one approach to choosing where to focus is based on analyzing the similarities and differences between programs and what metrics are being assessed to capitalize on impacting multiple programs.

The methodology of each program is extremely complex and may change, so refer to the details of each program's website to fully understand expectations. Based on Table 7.1, the domain that impacts most programs is infections, which may be referred to as the safety domain. Partnership for Patients, VBP, and HACRP all have financial incentives/penalties on the basis of performance. The methodological question is: how is performance compared? Is it based on performing better than a national rate, risk-adjusted rate, or a baseline of their own past performance? Additionally, the CMS Star Rating (Chapter 8) is a performance-based program and has infections as part of the safety domain. The main goal for the Partnership for Patients and HACRP is to reduce patient harm. For VBP, the premise is to improve care through comparing performance to a hospital's baseline performance while comparing to all hospitals. With the CMS Star Rating, performance is standardized to allow comparisons across domains and to a national rate.

CMS programs with a financial impact result in withholding a percentage of Medicare payments that tie incentives to performance. The payment a hospital

Table 7.1 Relationship between domains and programs

Domain	Partnership for Patients	P4P	VBP	HRRP	HACRP
Mortality			X		
Readmission	X			X	
Infections	X		X		X
Safety (PSI)			X		X
Patient experience		X	X		
Process		X	X		
Cost			X		

HACRP, Hospital-Acquired Condition Reduction Program; HRRP, Hospital Readmissions Reduction Program; P4P, Pay for Performance; PSI, VBP, Value-Based Purchasing.

receives is calculated through weighting various domains and metrics based on a performance criterion. While the metrics included within each program is subject to change, take a step back to think methodologically about an approach to handling these changes. Being proactive instead of reactive is the start of driving improvement efforts to hit those moving targets.

Infection/Safety Domain Methodology

Each of the programs (Partnership for Patients, VBP, HACRP, and CMS Star Rating) utilizes infection metrics. One common metric across all programs is CLABSI. Infection data is entered into the Centers for Disease Control and Prevention (CDC) using the National Healthcare Safety Network (NHSN). When reviewing NHSN, there are multiple different types of metrics available to analyze to help drive improvement efforts. It's important to step back and DEFINE all the available metrics to understand how each one contributes to the story. Within NHSN, four examples of metrics are available, and they are a CLABSI index, device utilization (DU) rate, standardized device utilization ratio (SUR), and a standardized infection ratio (SIR) (Table 7.2).

Each one of these metrics provides a different opportunity to tell a story. Think about how each of the metrics is defined and what it tells you about the story. Methodologically, think back to the statistics from Chapter 3 and what an index, rate, and ratio mean before jumping to conclusions and pay attention to the words preceding the index, rate, and ratio.

The CLABSI index in this context is not risk-adjusted. It is a measure of the total number of infections divided by patient care days and multiplied by 1,000. The interpretation of the index would be to indicate the number of infections per 1,000 patient care days. For example, a hospital having 5 infections and 2,500 patient care days would be equivalent to a 2.0 index. The DU rate for this infection is not risk-adjusted. It is calculated by dividing the total number of central line

Table 7.2 DEFINE tool for operationalizing CLABSI index metrics

DEFINE tool	Index	DU rate	SUR and SIR
Denominator	Patient care days	Patient care days	Expected index
Exclusion criteria	Varies based on the individual indicator		
Factor	Index multiplied by 1,000	Rate is multiplied by 100	Observed rate divided by expected rate
Inclusion criteria	Varies based on the individual indicator		
Numerator	Number of infections	Total line days	Observed index
Evaluate	Index is not risk-adjusted	Rate is not risk-adjusted	SIR is a risk-adjusted metric

CLABSI, central line-associated blood stream infection; DU, device utilization; SIR, standardized infection ratio; SUR, standardized utilization ratio.

days divided by patient care days and multiplied by 100. For example, 2,500 total patient care days divided by 3,000 line days would be a 0.83 device rate. A rate below 1 means that there are more line days than patient care days and rates above 1 indicate more patient care days than line days. The SUR and the SIR are both risk-adjusted and calculated as the observed rate divided by the expected rate. This expected rate is calculated utilizing a logistic regression model. For example, a 4.1 observed rate divided by a 3.6 expected rate equals a risk-adjusted ratio of 1.14. The interpretation of a ratio above 1.0 means performance is worse than expected and below 1.0 indicates performance is better than expected.

Depending on the program/initiative, NHSN provides these metrics using the CMS population or the entire patient population. A methodological approach to analyzing the operationalization of the provided statistics is the first step to understanding how each metric is utilized. New metrics and calculations may be available within NHSN, so refer to the CDC website (www.cdc.gov/nhsn/). After operationalizing the statistics, any uncertainty on where to focus is an opportunity to incorporate methodological thinking using the STOP tool to ask questions. When taking action to drive change, there is a difference between *thinking* and *doing*. Translating thoughts into actions is complicated. It is easy to think about reducing infections and ensuring there are 0 infections, but this is harder in practice. Developing unrealistic goals diminishes the effectiveness of being able to drive improvement (Muchinsky, 2006). A sample plan to reduce infections using the STOP tool is as follows:

- SMART goal: reduce CLABSI by 10% in 1 year.
- Think methodologically: develop checklist intervention to reduce infections.
- Operationalize: checklist must be defined by clinicians (i.e., using a focus group). Multiple metrics are used to drive change.
- Purpose: implement an evidence-based practice solution to reduce CLABSI.

The STOP planning tool provides a methodology to stimulate thinking and translate thoughts into actions that serve as a framework to determine next steps to guide the development of process metrics. This tool may provide an opportunity to think about the plan you want to accomplish or serve as a guide for what questions you should ask your clinical team to plan for success. The next phase is visually presenting the data. Trending existing data is an effective way to understand what happened in the past. what is currently happening in the present, and what will happen in the future.

Results

Trending the past and current data is critical to understanding how performance changes over time and tracking the success/failure of an intervention. Telling an effective story to drive future change involves utilizing a variety of statistics to better understand the big picture. Methodologically understanding the available data provides greater insight into assessing the intervention in multiple ways. The main focus of the initiatives (Partnership for Patients, VBP, HACRP, and CMS

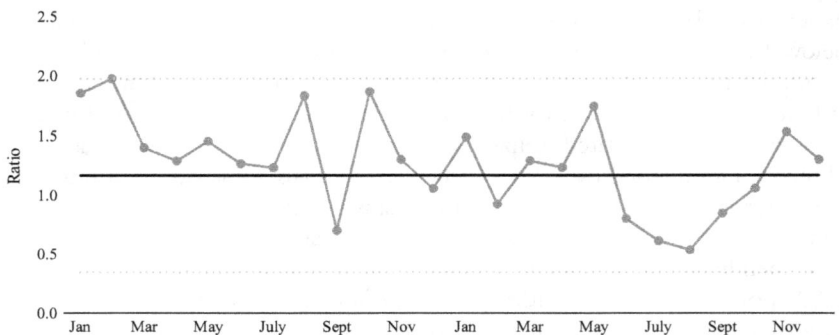

Figure 7.1 Central line–associated blood stream infection (CLABSI) index.

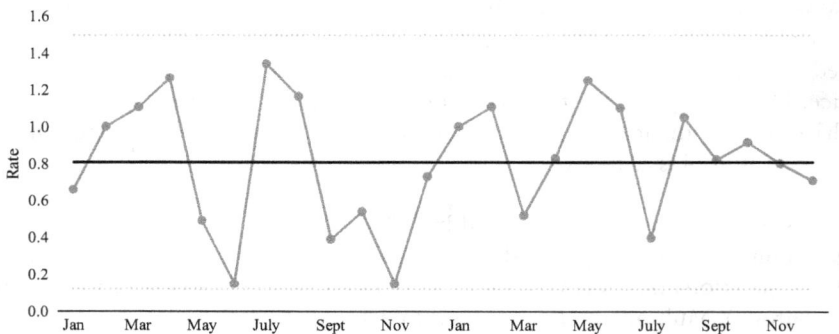

Figure 7.2 Central line–associated blood stream infection (CLABSI) device utilization rate.

Star Rating) may be on the CLABSI index, but this doesn't mean this is the only metric available to tell the story. There are additional metrics available within NHSN to enhance the story and drive change. The DU rate, SUR, and SIR are all trended along with the CLABSI index. Each component provides a different piece of the story.

Figures 7.1–7.4 all provide the trends from the past through the current. While one metric may result in financial penalties/incentives or performance, each of the metrics provides a unique perspective of the story to drive change. The CLABSI index (Figure 7.1) story revolves around the question, "how am I doing with respect to monthly infections?" The DU rate (Figure 7.2) focuses on trends of how often a central line is utilized in the hospital. Analyzing raw data is effective for knowing exactly how your hospital is performing. Focusing on only how your organization is performing only provides one side of the story. Move beyond the four walls of your organization and transition the question from, "how is my organization performing?" to "how do I compare to everyone else?" The only true way to know how you are doing is through benchmarking against

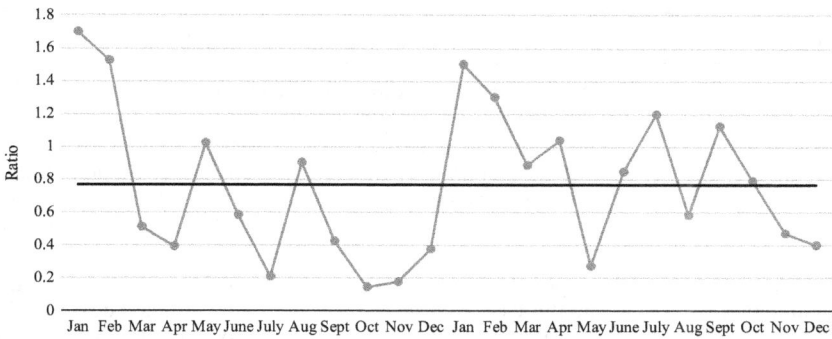

Figure 7.3 Central line-associated blood stream infection (CLABSI) standardized utilization ratio.

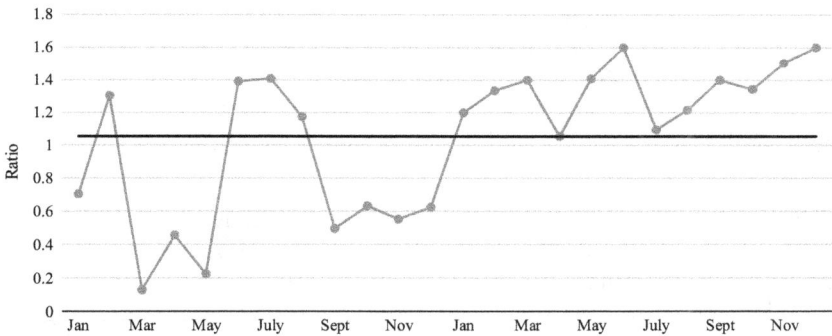

Figure 7.4 Central line-associated blood stream infection (CLABSI) standardized infection ratio.

others. However, if you only benchmark against others you may miss an opportunity to improve your raw metrics. The final two metrics, the SUR (Figure 7.3) and SIR (Figure 7.4), provide insight into how you are performing based on a statistical model.

The focus of the previous chapters was on using one or two metrics to analyze what happened and determining a path forward or utilizing the funnel-down approach from the big picture to actionable details. For this analysis, the goal is to analyze multiple interrelated metrics to understand the nuances between them and how they are combined together to tell the story. The DEFINE tool provides an overview of how each one of the metrics is measured. The next step is to focus on the FACTS of the individual metrics to identify statistical commonalities and differences between them to enhance the story.

Both Figures 7.1 and 7.2 are trended over time utilizing a control chart with 3 SD included on the graph. The DEFINE tool identified that these two metrics are both raw rates, so the story behind these metrics revolves around performance

Table 7.3 FACTS tool for index and rate

FACTS tool	CLABSI index	Device utilization rate
Formulas	Index = mean per month multiplied by 1,000 for index and by 100 for rate. Standard deviation	
Analyze patterns/ trends	Fluctuates with some data at the third standard deviation and some months trending down	Monthly data trends up and down with some points approaching 0%. Overall trend at the end appears to be trending down
Consider rules/ guidelines	One special cause variation above the third standard deviation. No other rule violations	Some data points close to the third standard deviation, but most variation is common cause
Think methodologically	Overall trend presents opportunity for improvement. Earlier months have a higher percentage of points above the mean. Later months have a dip, but an increase in index	Common cause variation presents an opportunity to examine process metrics. Pattern towards the end appears to be trending down
Statistics	Mean and standard deviation	

CLABSI, central line-associated blood stream infection.

in the current organization. Raw rates/indices are effective for monitoring trends within your organization, but provide limited insight into your performance with respect to others. Figures 7.3 and 7.4 contain risk-adjusted ratios utilizing a logistic regression model to calculate an expected standardized utilization (Figure 7.3) or standardized infection (Figure 7.4) to benchmark performance against others. Performance is trended utilizing a run chart.

Prior to analyzing the results to determine the story, take a step back and focus on the methodology, utilizing the FACTS tool for the index and rate (Table 7.3).

Analyzing the FACTS of what is presented in the control and run charts for the index and rate, respectively, leads down the path of being able to better understand the relationship between these two metrics. The CLABSI index focuses on the number of infections per patient care days. The interpretation of the patterns/ trends indicates whether or not infections are increasing or decreasing. Knowing the complexity of infections, one metric alone cannot tell the entire story. There are many **extraneous** and/or **confounding variables** (refer to Chapter 2) that can explain why a patient develops an infection and likely as many process metrics aimed at reducing infections. The DU rate is a measure of line days per patient care days. The probability or relationship of an infection occurring is greater when a central line is placed. A few questions to consider:

1. What does it mean when both the index and DU decrease? Is the decreased infection index a result of properly maintaining the central line or fewer patients having a central line?

2. What does it mean when the index increases, and the DU decreases? In this case, there are more infections, but fewer central lines. What would be the best approach to decrease infections?
3. What does it mean when the index decreases, and the DU increases? Is the decrease in index a result of using more devices? Could the volume of patients with a central line result in artificially decreasing the infections?

There are many different questions that can be asked when examining raw rates, such as the three scenarios posed above. Reacting to only an index or a rate may only tell part of the story. Another question to ask is how the performance of your organization compares to a statistical model.

Figures 7.3 and 7.4 provide risk-adjusted measures of DU and infection, respectively, utilizing run charts. The main goal of a risk-adjusted measure is to develop a statistical model that takes into consideration confounding variables that may influence the relationship between getting an infection or not, which is not possible when using the raw rate. The challenge with this is being able to identify and document these relationships. Regardless of this limitation, risk-adjusted metrics helps to eliminate potential issues of alternative explanations that are inherent in a raw index or rate.

Prior to analyzing where to improve or focus efforts, focus on the FACTS or the run charts (Table 7.4).

The FACTS of both the utilization (Figure 7.3) and infections (Figure 7.4) ratios provide a framework for how your organization is performing with respect to a statistical model. The ratios add a different perspective from what the index and rate provide. Let's ask the same questions as for the rate and index:

1. What does it mean when both the standardized utilization and infection ratios are decreasing? Does this mean that we are performing better than

Table 7.4 FACTS tool for ratios

FACTS tool	Standardized utilization ratio (SUR)	Standardized infection ratio (SIR)
Formulas	Ratio = observed rate divided by expected rate; mean = overall average for each metric. Logistic regression	
Analyze patterns/ trends	Variability in device utilization. One year consistently below 1, second year potential downward trend. Consistent high utilization in January and February	Variation in ratio. More data points below 1 in the first year, but second year has a consistent upward trend
Consider rules/ guidelines	No specific run chart interpretation guidelines are seen	More than 6 data points above the mean
Think methodologically	Ratios that are above 1.0 indicate performance is worse than expected and an index below 1.0 indicates performance is better than expected	
Statistics	Mean, standard deviation, logistic regression	

expected and utilizing fewer central lines or is the documentation of the patient's condition leading to a decrease or are we reducing the number of infections?

2. What does it mean if the utilization ratio decreases and the infection ratio increases? Are we utilizing central lines less, but the patient population with the central line is not expected to get an infection?

3. What does it mean if the utilization ratio increases and the infection ratio decreases? Are we using more central lines with a patient population that really needs a central line? Are the patients with a central line more complex?

What you won't know from the ratios is whether or not there are more infections within your organization. You only know whether you're performing better or worse than expected. This is the advantage of using multiple statistics, both risk-adjusted and raw rates when analyzing data.

The risk-adjusted metrics provide a benchmark to compare differences between what the observed value is and what the expected value should be. The result is that a ratio above 1.0 indicates performance is worse than expected and a ratio below 1.0 indicates performance is better than expected.

To compare and contrast the two ratios, let's look at a some different scenarios:

1. SIR above 1.0 and SUR at or below 1.0 means that there were more infections than expected, but less utilization of CLABSI. The interpretation could be that the number of device days for the current central lines is as expected or better than expected, but there is an issue with the lines that are placed as there are more infections.

2. SIR at or below 1.0 and SUR above 1.0 means there are more device days than expected, but fewer infections. The interpretation could be that the number of infections is better than expected, but the length of time a central line is in could be reduced.

3. Both raw metrics (index and rate) are decreasing, but the SIR and SUR are both above 1.0. The deceiving aspect of that scenario is that the raw rates in your organization are moving in the right direction. However, the model used to risk adjust the data indicates that more patients are getting infections and have central lines in longer than expected.

4. Both raw metrics (index and rate) are increasing, but the SIR and SUR are below 1.0. Even though there are more infections and longer central line days, the complexity of the patient population indicates that the organization is performing better than expected.

The moral of the story is that focusing on raw rates is effective for understanding how your organization is performing, but it does not take into consideration the complexity of the patient population. Risk adjustment provides a means for organizations to factor in confounding variables that have the potential to increase a patient's risk of infection.

The presented FACTS lay the groundwork for the final phase of developing a plan. The versatility of the STOP tool is incorporating methodological thinking after focusing on the FACTS to direct targeted thinking or pose critical questions for the future as improvements benefit from a clear focus on where to go next. A properly thought-out plan is the difference between success and failure, so invest the time to avoid jumping to conclusions or relying on hunches or beliefs. A revisit of the STOP tool following a focus on the FACTS resulted in greater clarity towards improvement. This revised STOP plan is focused less on a reduction of infections, but rather on the variation in trends and incorporation of multiple metrics to create a plan around improving process metrics.

- SMART goal – ensure consistent evidence-based processes to reduce infections within 1 year.
- Think – conduct focus groups with clinicians to understand the clinical steps followed to prevent infection.
- Operationalize – determine the individual process metric definitions to develop valid and reliable ways of measuring performance; for example, using the index and device days.
- Purpose – ensure consistent processes are put in place that result in a decreased variability.

Discussion

Driving sustainable change to move a metric is no small feat. Focusing on one metric when there are many variables that explain a relationship is not ideal for understanding where to focus or what to focus on. This is also true with the various programs/initiatives that hospitals are being held accountable for. The question regarding where to focus is not an easy answer. For example, focusing on the CLABSI SIR because it's included in specific programs and ignoring the index, DU rate, or the SUR could lead to mixed messages. Throughout this chapter, the recommendation was to methodologically review all programs/initiatives to better understand the metrics that are associated with each one. It is not uncommon for multiple programs/initiatives to utilize similar metrics, so a question of where to focus may lead you down the path to improve one metric that impacts multiple programs. In the case of infections, taking advantage of multiple metrics provides more of the story.

Healthcare professionals focus on solving the right problem but may often ask the wrong questions or utilize one metric to make a decision. Having a predetermined path towards improvement is not always an effective avenue to drive improvement. Where you want to be may differ from where you should be. Don't mistake one fork in the path as a definitive solution towards moving forward. When beginning the process of analyzing metrics, it's not only important to leverage the statistics, but also to take into consideration the past, present, and future. Healthcare organizations are not always in the position to directly influence future government initiatives, but remaining proactive and involved can pave the way for the future by forming advocacy groups or partnering with other organizations that strive to change the way healthcare is delivered. The best way to plan for the future is to focus on the past, track the present, and be versatile to changes in approaching the future. Initiatives change, so knowing what metrics impact which program/initiatives will allow you to hit those moving targets.

Monitoring patterns and trends within data is effectively done through run charts and control charts, but they are not the only means for visually displaying a story. Any graphical representation of data must effectively display the past and present to provide support for changing the future. The bigger question is how to effectively manage change and influence behavior to ensure consistent future practices. The pathway to improvement does not happen overnight. Understanding barriers to change or resistors to change is equally as important as implementing an intervention focused on improving process and outcome metrics. As with any government initiative and evolution of healthcare, change will occur. Sometimes change is driven based on evolution in research, advances in technology, or political leadership. The focus of the future is uncertain, but one thing that will happen is change. How we react and respond to change is an important factor for successfully implementing a sustainable intervention.

Not everyone responds to change in the same way, so don't expect an intervention to solve all problems. There will be those individuals who quickly adopt an intervention and others who resist change. No matter how much planning and thinking is put in place, barriers that impact the successful implementation of an intervention still exist. Sometimes these barriers are alleviated with the implementation of a methodological and statistical approach and other times there are factors beyond our control, such as other initiatives/variables occurring at the same time or personal factors related to an individual. The question is whether or not change is a result of the employee or the leader. Whenever initiating change, it's critically important to focus on not only the present, but how past behavior impacts future performance. Proper tools help with guiding future directions and align thinking to ensure a methodological approach is consistently followed. Three tools are available to assist in this process:

1. DEFINE your metrics.
2. Focus on the FACTS.
3. STOP and ask questions.

When developing behavioral interventions, there will likely be resistors to change where some factors cannot be controlled as they are related to events surrounding the intervention or individual factors. From a methodological perspective, there is a concern when other reasons explain a change in behavior that is separate from the intervention (internal validity). For example, hospital priorities for treating sepsis patients prior to the implementation of the CMS requirements for sepsis reporting may change how an organization focuses on improving sepsis outcomes. Financial reimbursement/penalty for specific metrics may change the focus as well. Multiple initiatives are implemented at the same time, so pinpointing change due to one particular intervention may not be possible. These variables are

referred to as confounding or extraneous variables and methodologically the goal
is to reduce them as much as possible.

Resistors to Change

The other barriers to effective implementation originate from individuals. There
are many factors as to why an individual would resist change. Within Chapter 1
there was a discussion on placing individuals into different groups based on
adoption of change. Two of these groups were discussed: early adopters (those
quick to adopt change) and laggards (those slow to adopt change) (Rogers, 2010).
The remaining groups are innovators, early majority, and late majority. As part of
Rogers' (2010) work, the categories of change is a result of a theory known as
"diffusion of innovation," which discusses how, why, and how quickly/slowly new
ideas affect change. Based on the theory, a bell curve was created to indicate the
frequency of which different groups of individuals adopt change (Figure 7.5). The
innovators account for 2.5% of the share of individuals adopting change. The early
adopters and innovators combined account for between 16% (2.5% and 13.5%,
respectively). Change takes time and by the late majority, there are still 50% of
individuals late to adopt change.

Overcoming barriers/resistors to change is a key component to the successful
implementation and adoption of an intervention. The time lapse between each
category of adopter varies based on the initiative. Change is a continuous process, but persistence and dedication to change along with time make the difference between success and failure. Knowing and understanding the population of
interest provide insight into effective means for implementing change. A rarely
disputed fact is data. However, there are those individuals who will debate and
dispute the validity of the data or determine alternative explanations to discount
the story. It is incredibly hard to discount the presented facts, assuming the methodology applied is rigorous. This is one reason why focusing on the past and
present and understanding the future guided by a methodological approach to
implementing behavioral-based interventions is an effective means of achieving
those moving targets and overcoming barriers to change.

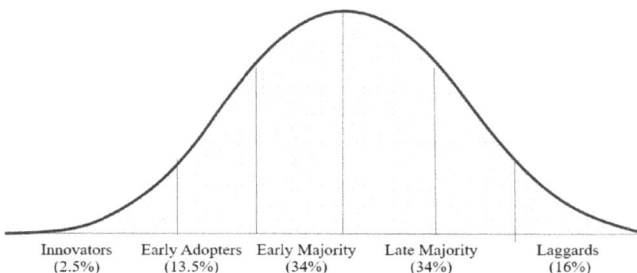

| Innovators | Early Adopters | Early Majority | Late Majority | Laggards |
| (2.5%) | (13.5%) | (34%) | (34%) | (16%) |

Figure 7.5 Normal distribution of change.

Discussion Questions

- What methods do you use to keep a pulse on not only what's happening within your organization? How do you leverage what you know outside your four walls to drive change?
- How do performance-based incentive/penalty programs impact organizational goals?
- When deciding what metrics to focus on, what methods do you use to determine where to improve? Performance-based metrics impacting multiple programs? Priorities of the health of the community?
- Have you ever focused on the right problem, but asked the wrong question or focused on the wrong problem, but asked the right question?
- If hindsight is 20/20, then how would you utilize existing knowledge of governmental programs to change how you address a problem in the future?
- How do you overcome barriers to those resisting change to encourage them to get on board with your intervention or plan to improve the healthcare delivery process?
- When implementing change, how do you identify and convince key stake holders to focus on your improvement effort and how do you encourage individuals to adopt this change?
    - How do you overcome those individuals who may continually look for a means to discredit the results you're presenting to fit the vision of how they see the story behind what is happening?

8   CMS Star Rating

"If at first you don't succeed, fix the process and reach for the stars."

Introduction

Focusing on the four walls within a healthcare organization is no longer sustainable. There is intense competition stemming not only from competing hospitals, but also securing alliances with ambulatory hospitals and physician office practices to generate income and competing with other hospitals across the country based on financial/performance incentives/penalties set by Centers for Medicare/Medicaid Services (CMS) and other regulatory/governmental initiatives. It is advantageous to inquire with others outside your organization to have a complete picture of what is happening and how comparisons are being made to ensure effective improvement efforts inside the four walls. There is increasing pressure from regulatory and governmental agencies to not only improve patient outcomes, but focus on the entire continuum of care or deal with financial penalties. One particular initiative, the High Value Healthcare Collaborative (HVHC), focuses on sharing and streamlining best practices across the country to drive policy decisions.

Healthcare organizations must transform into high-quality service organizations as they are scrutinized for patient outcomes based on rankings, not only internal to their organization, but across the world. Patients are more educated and technologically savvy, and desire high-quality outcomes and exceptional healthcare experience in a timely and accurate manner. As consumers of information, patients research the place they may choose to receive care. Patients have expectations to receive high-quality, top-notch care with superb outcomes and utilize data to make informed choices. To put into perspective, consider these facts from the American Hospital Association (AHA): there are over 6,100 hospitals in the United States with more than 924,000 beds and 36,000,000 hospital admissions totaling expenses over $1,112,000,000,000 (www.aha.org/research/rc/stat-studies/fast-facts.shtml). These hospitals generate both qualitative and quantitative data on every patient, to the extent that experts estimate a new patient generates 4 megabytes a year and each subsequent year, leading to terabytes of data waiting to be analyzed (www.nextech.com/blog/healthcare-data-growth-an-exponential-problem).

This data is converted into measures not only utilized for making decisions to drive patient outcomes, but also to rate hospitals. These measures are not always new, as some measures may appear in multiple programs/initiatives. Hospital ratings are published for the public to view in places like U.S. News and World Report, Leapfrog, Top Doctors, Healthgrades, etc. An online search of "compare doctors" leads to hits like www.zocdoc.com, www.medicare.gov/physiciancompare, www. healthgrades.com, www.1800doctors.com, www.consumerreports.org, www. ucomparehealthcare.com, www.webmd.com, and www.vitals.com that allow for comparisons of physicians across a variety of metrics. Although there may be disagreement with the results, websites like these exist and patients may use them to make decisions regardless of their accuracy.

Not only is it possible to compare healthcare providers and hospitals, but organizations are leveraging research methodological designs and statistical models to standardize metrics for the purposes of comparing performance across hospitals. Governmental and private organizations are analyzing data to develop benchmarks for comparative purposes. CMS has one methodology to compare ratings of hospitals posted publicly for review. This methodology led to the development of a star rating comprised of 50+ metrics categorized into domains that are grouped into one score where each hospital receives a 1–5-star rating. The Leapfrog Group is another organization comparing hospitals on a variety of metrics using voluntarily reported data with a disclaimer of not being liable for implications from decisions made using their data. Hospital ratings are, and continue to be, publicly available for patients to evaluate hospital performance. Knowing the data source, methodology to collect this data, and statistical model becomes critical to understanding the validity of the results. Leapfrog relies on self-report with data validation built in and the CMS Star Rating is based on administrative claims data. The CMS Star Rating is complex and warrants a further discussion on the methodology and statistics behind the meaning of what a "star" is.

First and foremost, there has been a debate around the methodology of the star rating. Take, for example, the letter from the AHA regarding the statistical model surrounding the calculation of the CMS Star Rating (www.aha.org/ advocacy-issues/letter/2017/170925-let-thompson-cms-star-ratings.pdf).   The details contained within the letter are statistically and methodologically sound and provide recommendations for improvement. The transparency of the methodology and model behind the CMS Star Rating provides an opportunity for being proactive and reacting to the information in a methodological way. CMS has taken into consideration this feedback and altered their statistical model beginning with the December 2017 release. It is also likely that additional feedback will be incorporated in future releases.

Composite and Summary Scores

The overall idea of condensing multiple measures into one overall score is not new. Agency for Healthcare Research and Quality (AHRQ) discussed composite scores and summary scores as two methodologies for combining multiple measures (www.ahrq.gov/professionals/quality-patient-safety/talkingquality/create/ scores/combinemeasures.html). The differentiating factor between a composite and summary score is the relationship between the metrics. When metrics are highly related to each other a composite score is calculated. For example, patient satisfaction measures are considered composite scores because they all measure an aspect of patient satisfaction. A summary score is calculated when the desire is to calculate one score for multiple metrics that are not highly related to each other. For example, combining multiple measures on a variety of different performance dimensions (i.e., mortality, readmission, cost, median wait time in the emergency department, efficiency of imaging, infection, etc.) to determine an overall score representing performance.

The only nuance between a summary or composite score is on the basis of the combined metrics being correlated to each other and may come down to a matter of semantics. Regardless of whether or not a score is referred to as a composite or a summary, the desire of creating an easy-to-interpret metric that captures the quality of care being delivered is important. Choosing a hospital that expresses the needs and preferences of a patient is a difficult and personal decision. Having one metric to evaluate performance is much less cognitively burdensome for patients than focusing on 50+ metrics when they may not be familiar with all the medical jargon.

Process and Outcome Metrics

CMS Hospital Compare (Chapter 9) created a comparison tool summarizing over 50 measures into an overall hospital rating for patients to make informed decisions on which hospital is right for their needs. Hospital Compare shows how hospitals over the country have treated conditions compared to the national average and uses a star rating as a measure of overall performance. The star rating is an analytical model developed using CMS data to compare hospitals by awarding a maximum of 5 stars. A 1 star indicates an organization with "much below average quality," while a 5 star indicates an organization with "well above average quality." Like any methodology, the number and type of metrics may change, so visit the CMS website for the most up-to-date information (www.medicare.gov/hospitalcompare/Data/Data-Updated.html#).

Now why would CMS provide one overall star rating as an indicator for hospital performance using more than 50 metrics? One response is, why not publicly post all steps in a surgery instead of the overall mortality rate? Outcome measures in general represent the end result of a process. Arriving at that result is complex, because multiple process metrics influence the outcome. The outcome should not be the gold standard for performance, because the process is as important as the outcome. Without a well-defined and structured process, the outcome may lack consistency. Lack of consistency (reliability) increases variations in practice, which could cause variations in outcome. An opportunity exists to develop protocols and processes to ensure consistent performance. Since many processes impact one outcome, focusing only on the outcome is a missed opportunity. Process metrics provide an opportunity to determine actions requiring change to improve that desired outcome (Rubin, Pronovost, & Diette, 2001). Do you have any interest in knowing all the steps a pastry chef goes through to create pastries or only care that it tastes/looks good? The point is the brain is limited to the amount of information (i.e., up to around seven pieces of information) consumed at one time, which may be a reason for focusing on one outcome metric instead of many process or outcome metrics (Miller, 1956). This makes it overwhelming to nearly impossible for anyone to focus on over 50 different metrics concurrently, hence the ease of interpretation for a star rating.

Before detailing the nuances of the star methodology, it's important to take a step back and DEFINE the population, focus on the FACTS, then STOP to ask questions. The DEFINE tool is versatile by forcing a methodological approach to understand a measure at a high level or the construct validity of an individual metric. Jumping to conclusions to fix a problem not fully understood will not result in improvement. Likewise, fixing an outcome metric without understanding the process will not result in improvement. Take time to focus on the method- ology of what is presented and the statistics calculated to maximize the interpret- ation of the data. Know that it is not possible to solve everything, so inquire with others to have a complete picture of what is happening and how to improve.

CMS Star Rating Methodology

The CMS Star Rating consists of seven domains and up to 60 measures where four domains are weighted 22% and three are weighted 4% with weights, measures, and domains being subject to change. The purpose of weighting metrics is to ensure certain metrics have a stronger influence on the overall star rating. The seven domains are as follows: mortality, safety, readmission, patient experience, effective- ness of care, timeliness of care, and efficient use of medical imaging. To determine an appropriate direction to improve, it's important to focus on defining the popu- lation of these metrics (Table 8.1).

Every approach to an analysis must begin with examining the research meth- odology and statistics behind the program/measure. The DEFINE tool identi- fied metrics measured as rates, indices, ratios, average minutes, risk-adjusted rates/ indices, and composite metrics. Prior to the analysis, the DEFINE tool highlighted the importance of external validity and construct validity questions to ask based on the information obtained. The external validity arises from how the data is generalized (external validity) between patient populations (i.e., Medicare patients to all patients) and how each domain is operationalized (construct validity).

External Validity

Some metrics focus on inpatient, outpatient, and/or Medicare patients. While care shouldn't depend on the type of patient (Medicare or not), knowing certain patients are included in the metrics is an important consideration when general- izing the results (i.e., external validity). When an analysis is conducted on a sample of the population, confidence intervals are provided to generalize results from the sample (i.e., Medicare) to the population (i.e., all patients). The DEFINE tool is a systematic methodology to better understand the population being measured. Discounting or poking holes in results utilizing Medicare patients because an organization provides care for all types of patients doesn't fix the problem or

Table 8.1 Star domain definitions

DEFINE tool	Patient experience	Timeliness of care	Efficient use of medical imaging	Mortality	Safety	Readmission	Effectiveness of care
Denominator	All inpatient	All outpatient	Medicare outpatient	Medicare inpatient	All inpatient or Medicare inpatient	Medicare inpatient	All inpatient and/or outpatient
Exclusion criteria	Varies by metric						
Factor	Rate	Minutes	Rate	Risk-adjusted rate	Risk-adjusted rate/ratio and composite	Risk-adjusted rate	Rate
Inclusion criteria	All inpatient	All outpatient	Medicare outpatient	ICD codes vary by metric, Medicare inpatient	ICD codes vary by metric, all inpatient or Medicare inpatient	ICD codes vary by metric, Medicare inpatient	All inpatient and/or outpatient
Numerator	Survey top-box responses	Patients meeting criteria for inclusion		Patient expirations based on inclusion criteria	Patients with complication, infections that meet inclusion criteria	Patient readmissions based on inclusion criteria	Patients meeting criteria for inclusion
Evaluate			Understanding how patients are included assists in providing direction on where to focus				

ICD, *International Classification of Diseases*.

change the outcome (i.e., star rating). Think about transitioning action to be proactive instead of reactive through the following:

1. Utilize methodological and statistical knowledge to influence/challenge the methodology of the statistical analysis (i.e., AHA's letter to CMS regarding the star rating).
2. Alternatively, be proactive through reframing the question and asking how departments are improving specific patient outcomes through process improvement.

Construct Validity

Generalizing results from one situation to another is not the only issue. Metrics found within the literature and defined by various healthcare/government organizations may be different. Metrics are created and definitions defended regularly. Properly operationalizing metrics enhances the validity of the results by allowing everyone to know exactly how a particular metric is measured. Leverage the DEFINE tool to identify how domains and metrics are assessed. Starting with the concept of a rate, Chapter 1 discussed rates as being an observed or risk-adjusted rate. The definition of a "rate" has different interpretations based on the definition. An observed mortality rate of 1.5% is different from a risk-adjusted rate of 1.5%. A 1.5% mortality rate indicates that, out of all patients discharged from the hospital, 1.5% of them expired. A risk-adjusted rate of 1.5% is calculated using a logistic regression model where variables influencing the outcome are included in a model to predict a mortality rate. Prior to making improvements, utilize the DEFINE tool for operationalizing individual metrics within a domain (Table 8.2).

Table 8.2 DEFINE tool for stroke mortality

DEFINE tool	MORT-30-STK: *acute ischemic stroke 30-day rate*
Denominator	Medicare patients 65 years old or older with an initial index hospitalization for a principal diagnosis of ischemic stroke
Exclusion criteria	Denominator – patients leaving against medical advice, transfers from another acute care facility, unreliable data, enrolled in Medicare hospice or Medicare 12 months prior to hospitalization
Factor	Risk-adjusted using a logistic regression model with muliple variables
Inclusion criteria	Initial index admission for a specific diagnosis code of ischemic stroke (ICD codes)
Numerator	All-cause patient expirations up to 30 days after discharge
Evaluate	30-day post-hospitalization all-cause risk-adjusted mortality rate for the Medicare population with an index hospitalization for a primary diagnosis of ischemic stroke. Model adjusted for multiple clinical variables

ICD, *International Classification of Diseases.*

Statistical Concepts

The CMS Star Rating is a calculation of statistical concepts (i.e., rates, indices, standardized infection ratios, average minutes, and risk-adjusted rates). The DEFINE tool is versatile with its methodological ability to break down statistical concepts to understand the calculations, operationalize domains, and systematically evaluate how metrics are calculated. The following list highlights some calculations or factors within the star rating.

- *Rates* – the sum of the numerator divided by the sum of the denominator multiplied by 100.
- *Indices* – this varies based on the metric. Sum of the numerator divided by sum of the denominator multiplied by 1,000 or an observed rate divided by expected rate.
- *Standardized infection ratios* – observed infection rates divided by expected infection rates. Expected infection rate is based on a logistic regression model.
- *Average minutes* – emergency department measures based on time to achieve a metric.
- *Risk-adjusted rates* – a logistic regression model used to control for variables and calculate a rate.

The statistics are converted into z-scores, confidence intervals, and percentiles. Interpreting all these statistics is a challenge, because the direction for improved performance varies based on the analyzed metric. For example, the safety domain consists of a standardized infection ratio where a ratio below 1 is better; the patient experience domain results in high individual rates where higher scores are better; and the mortality domain has risk-adjusted rates that are typically low where lower scores are better. As a result, the safety domain measure of 0.61, patient experience domain measure of 92, and a mortality domain measure of 7% are all calculated using different statistics and scales of measurement.

The first statistic is the z-score. From a statistical perspective, a **z-score distribution** standardizes data using the following formula: $z = (\text{mean} - \text{mu})/\text{sigma}$. In other words, calculating a z-score requires the sample average (mean), population average (mu), and population standard deviation (sigma). A z-score distribution converts data from any scale of measurement into the same scale. This means that the interpretation of a z-score $= 1$ is the same for patient experience, mortality, and safety. It is not necessary to remember what direction results in improved performance. An added benefit of a z-score for all metrics is the ability to combine z-scores into one metric (i.e., one star rating).

The next statistical concept is the **confidence interval**. Confidence intervals are helpful when a sample of data is analyzed with the intention of generalizing to the larger population. Confidence intervals are calculated using 90%, 95%, or 99% to state how confident the results of the population value will fall within the interval (Figure 8.1). The 95% confidence interval is the most common. As the confidence increases (i.e., 90% to 95% to 99%), the interval becomes larger. CMS utilizes confidence intervals to estimate what the population value would

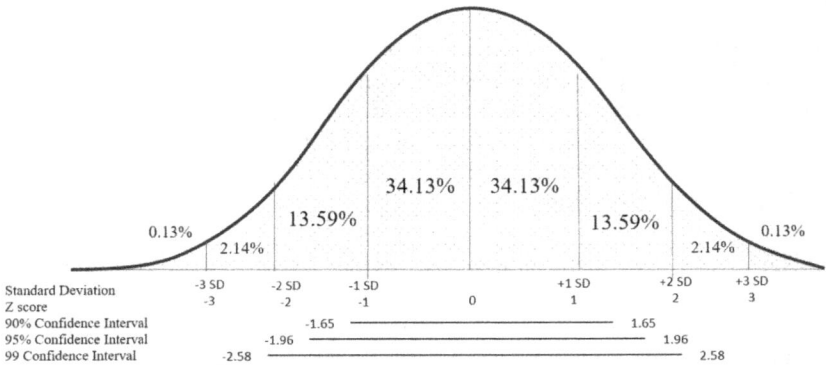

Figure 8.1 Bell-shape curve with confidence intervals.

Box 8.1 An Inherent Benchmark: Decoding Intelligence Quotient (IQ) Scores One Z-Score at a Time

IQ is used to measure intelligence through mathematical ability, spatial ability, etc. Using a z-score distribution provides a frame of reference and an internal benchmark through displaying data on a bell-shaped curve. This means within 1 SD, or 1 z-score, ~67% of the population is captured, within 2 SD captures ~95% and 3 SD capture ~99%. All this information translates into raw scores where a z-score of 0 is equal to a raw IQ score of 100 and population standard deviation of 15. A z-score of −1 to 1 corresponds to a raw IQ score of 85–115, which is calculated by either adding or subtracting the population standard deviation. Think about it next time when someone states their IQ is 140. A little math reveals an IQ of 140 is beyond 2 SD or above a 2.0 z-score. To take it one step further, there are tables available that convert z-scores into probabilities. The 2.0 z-score converts to a probability of 0.0228 or 2.28%. This means that there is a 2.28% chance of an individual having an IQ of 140.

---

be from the analysis. The reason a confidence interval is used is because the mortality domain, for example, consists of Medicare patients. Hospitals treat all patients, so a Medicare mortality rate is used as a sample with a 95% confidence interval calculated to determine what the hospital mortality rate may be. This confidence interval is utilized to determine if a hospital is performing better than the national rate (i.e., the entire confidence interval is above the national rate), worse than the national rate (i.e., the entire confidence interval is below the national rate), or the same as the national rate (i.e., the confidence interval contains the national rate).

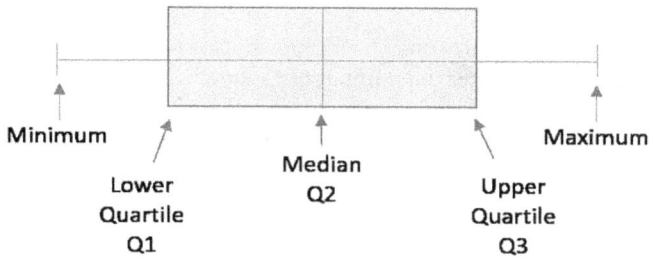

Figure 8.2 Box-and-whiskers plot.

The final statistical concept in the star rating are percentiles. Percentiles are utilized to demonstrate performance of an individual hospital within the larger comparative database. Recall from Chapter 3 the mean, median, and mode are measures of central tendency or measures of variability. A percentile is an additional measure of variability that structures the data to determine values that would fall above or below a particular score. For example, the 50th percentile is the same as the median in that 50% of scores fall above and below that value. The most common percentiles are the 25th, 50th, and 75th percentile. Some organizations provide a top decile or the top 10% of performers, which is equivalent to the 90th percentile. Percentiles allow an organization to know where they stand with respect to everyone else.

Confidence intervals and percentiles are graphically presented utilizing a box-and-whiskers plot to more effectively tell the story. A box-and-whiskers plot (Figure 8.2) is created to depict outliers and show the distribution of all data. The "box" corresponds to percentiles and the "whiskers" reflect the confidence interval. The middle of the box is the 50th percentile and the top and bottom line of the box represent the 25th and 75th percentile, respectively. The whiskers typically represent the 95% confidence interval, but other confidence intervals may be utilized.

CMS Star Statistical Methodology

The star statistical methodology is complex. Those interested in the details of the statistical methodology are advised to review the information available on the CMS website. The following discussion is intended to provide a high-level overview of the statistical methods of the star rating. In December 2017, the statistical methodology was changed, so it is possible that future releases of the star rating may result in slight variations of the statistical methodology utilized to assign a star on the basis of weights, metrics, or modifications in the statistical model. Hospitals are provided an overall star rating assuming they have a minimum of three of the seven domains and are measured on average using 39 measures with a minimum of nine and a maximum of ~60, which may change in the future to be inclusive of more metrics.

K-Means Clustering

The culmination of all statistics into one star rating is accomplished through K-means clustering, where "K" indicates the number of groups. In the case of the CMS Star Rating, the "K" is 5 based on an individual hospital receiving 1–5 stars. The methodology provided for the star rating is identified as a six-step process (www. Qualitynet.org). The six-step process is clearly detailed, but our goal was to simplify the complexity of the model through discussing the statistical aspects in three steps. The overall methodology behind this statistical technique is to utilize z-scores to aggregate metrics into one overall score using three statistically complex steps:

1.   Conversion of raw scores into z-scores
2.   Latent variable modeling
3.   K-means clustering.

Step 1: Conversion of Raw Score into z-Scores

The statistical model utilizes z-scores to combine all metrics into a single measure. The first step is to convert all raw scores into an equivalent z-score. The purpose is to ensure that the distributions of data measured on different scales of measurement are equal. For example, it is not feasible to compare the influence of a mortality rate in the single digits, patient satisfaction measures between 70% and 90%, or a standardized infection ratio of below 1. Recall the interpretation of a standard normal distribution and that 3 SD capture ~99% of variability and 2 SD capture ~95% of variability. This means a z-score between −3 and 3 captures ~99% of variability for all metrics. The distribution of a bell-shaped curve or normal distribution forces the majority of organizations in the middle of the distribution. In other words, statistically 68% of hospitals will be a 3-star hospital. The caveat to this statement is that a statistical methodology smooths out the distribution, resulting in more opportunities for a hospital to be a 3-, 4-, or 5-star. To add to the complexity, performance metrics are moving targets, so while your organization improves, others are improving as well. This means an organization scoring below the national rate would have to improve at a faster rate than the entire nation. This improvement is included in the calculations of the nationwide rates, which makes the moving target change during every release.

Converting raw scores into z-scores requires three pieces of information: the sample average, population average, and population standard deviation. The publicly available CMS dataset provides population averages and standard deviations, then a formula converts the raw score into a z-score. Now all metrics, regardless of the scale of measurement, are measured on the same scale to compare across metrics/domains. The same method to convert a raw value to a z-score will also convert a z-score to a raw value. This is helpful when Hospital Compare provides a standard score or z-score mortality. A mortality rate with a z-score of 1.3 provides some insight, but taking action from a rate is more intuitive than a z-score. For example, improving a mortality z-score of 1.3 is different than reducing an 11.2% mortality rate.

Box 8.2 The Philosophy of Mortality

Not to be philosophical, but stop and think about what mortality is and what it means to measure it. Looking up "mortality" in a dictionary results in five definitions according to www.dictionary.com:

1. The state or condition of being subject to death
2. Relative frequency of deaths in a specific population
3. Mortal beings, collectively
4. Death or destruction on a large scale, as from war, plague, or famine
5. Obsolete.

Mortality may have multiple meanings, which is where the operationalization of how it is being measured is critical. Utilizing the DEFINE tool provides a methodological framework for developing a definition to observe or measure the metric. This converts the word mortality from a latent variable to a measured variable when a definition is added to clarify how to measure it.

Step 2: Statistical Technique: Latent Variable Modeling

Building a model involves examining a group of variables that explain a particular relationship of interest. In this case, the goal is to determine overall performance for an organization on the basis of 50+ measures grouped into higher-level domains. There are multiple ways to build a model, such as a logistic regression model or latent variable modeling. Beginning with logistic regression, it is a statistical technique used to make a prediction for a specific outcome (i.e., mortality, readmission, infection, etc.) while controlling for other variables (i.e., age, comorbidities, etc.) influencing the outcome. Doing this allows comparison of mortality rates across organizations regardless of the patient population, because the logistic regression provides risk-adjusted mortality rates. Star ratings require different calculations, because the predicted outcome is not directly observable (what does a star mean?).

Logistic regression is similar to latent variable modeling except the goal is to predict a latent variable. Methodologically, a **latent variable** (mortality domain or star rating) cannot be directly observed or measured, but **manifest variables** (acute myocardial infarction (AMI) mortality, chronic obstructive pulmonary disease mortality, stroke mortality, death due to complications) are used as proxy variables to calculate a domain score or star rating. Logistic regression predicts an observable criterion variable (i.e., overall mortality rates). Latent variable modeling predicts an unobservable variable (i.e., a star rating or an aggregate mortality domain comprised of multiple disease-specific mortality rates). The seven domains of the CMS Star Rating (mortality, safety of care, readmission, patient experience, effectiveness of care, timeliness of care, and efficient use of medical imaging) are constructs that cannot be directly observed or measured, but are operationalized

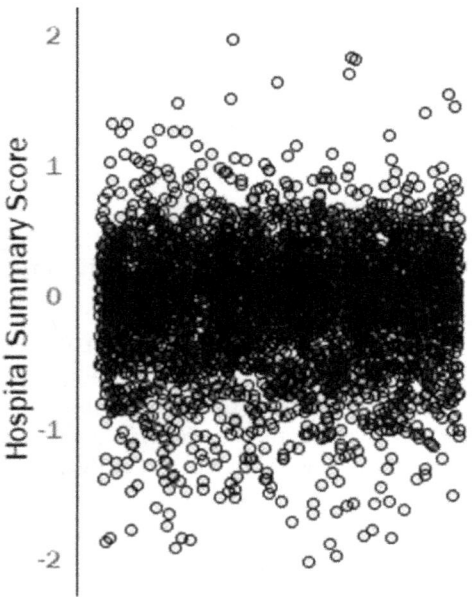

Figure 8.3 Scatter plot.
Source: Healthcare Association of New York State, 2017.

by calculating observable metrics. Now you may be thinking, "I can measure mortality!" and that would be right. That statement provides context on how to DEFINE a metric to be able to measure it. Asking the question, "I want to know what my heart failure mortality rate is" converts the latent construct into an observable measure.

The advantage of using latent variable modeling is the ability to account for hospitals with missing information, variability in how data is reported to CMS, adding or removing metrics over time, and examining relationships between metrics falling within a particular domain, which logistic regression cannot do. The end result of a latent variable model provides a wealth of information regarding how much influence or weight, which is known as a **factor loading**, a particular metric has on the overall domain. Metrics with low weights are evaluated to determine whether or not they should be removed from the model. The development of a model results in the calculation of scores that can then be graphically displayed through a scatter plot or scatter diagram (Figure 8.3).

Step 3: K-Means Clustering

The results of the scatter plot are analyzed through a clustering technique that groups the data together for ease of interpretation. One statistical technique for analyzing clusters of data is called K-means clustering; this utilizes latent variable modeling to condense scores into groups or K-means where the "K" indicates

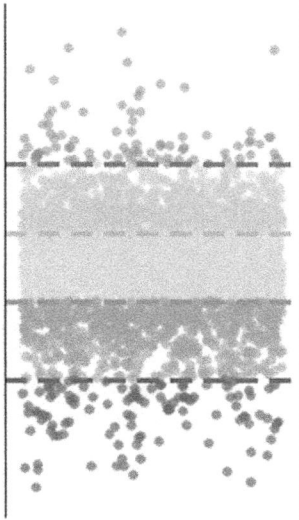

Figure 8.4 K-means clustering.
Source: Healthcare Association of New York State, 2017.

the number of desired groups (Figure 8.4). The statistical calculations behind the scenes involve a weighted average of the latent variable model to then predict a star rating through combining the latent variables or measure domains (i.e., mortality domain, patient experience domain, etc.). Each break in the line on Figure 8.4 is considered a cutoff score required in order to fall within that particular group. While the star rating results in one overall star, from a statistical perspective each individual domain has the potential of being assigned a star.

Box-and-Whiskers Plot

The last methodological component of analyzing statistics involves the box-and-whiskers plot. A box-and-whiskers plot utilizes confidence intervals and percentiles to provide an interpretation of performance relative to others in the dataset. Step back and focus on the FACTS and statistical concepts in the box-and-whiskers plot. Within the graphical representation of the box-and-whiskers plot (Figure 8.5), the box displays the 25th, 50th, and 75th percentile, the whiskers displays a 90%, 95%, or 99% confidence interval, and any data point beyond the whisker is an outlier. The interpretation for the 75th percentile (or box) indicates that the organization is performing better than 75% of others within the entire dataset or that 25% of organizations are performing better. The confidence interval provides the spread of data points in the dataset. A 95% confidence interval indicates that 95% of all data points fall within the range (or whiskers) on the graph. The wider the percentile (box) or confidence interval (whiskers), the more variability on a given metric.

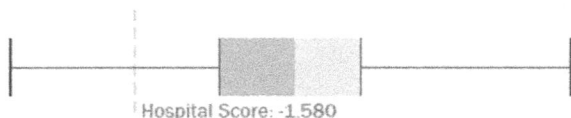

Hospital Score: -1.580

Figure 8.5 Box-and-whiskers plot.
Source: Healthcare Association of New York State, 2017.

Results

With an understanding of the research methodology behind the CMS Star Rating and statistical concepts utilized, the next step is graphically representing data to effectively tell a story to improve. Turning all this data into a comprehensive story to convey a particular message is complicated, let alone combine the sevendomains with 50+ metrics from all of the CMS data into a single star rating. Utilize the funnel-down approach and focus on the overall star rating and work backwards. The funnel-down approach starts with a high-level analysis to provide a summary or outline of the analytics and proceeds towards the detail to determine where to focus.

The star rating story is told through a dashboard developed by Healthcare Association of New York State (HANYS) and is used with their permission. Their comprehensive dashboard provides an easy-to-interpret analytic story of how to leverage outside data to benchmark your individual organization. A 3-star hospital is utilized to illustrate the story utilizing the funnel-down approach (see Chapter 6). Keep in mind that 3 stars is the overall performance rating, but this does not mean all domains result in a 3-star rating.

When all hospitals are plotted on a distribution, the result is the hospital summary score in Figure 8.4 where the entire distribution of hospitals is broken into 5-star categories using the K-means clustering technique. The dashed lines indicate the cutoff scores between stars. Movement into a higher/lower star rating is more likely for hospitals near these lines. Step back and take a methodological approach to interpreting the CMS Star Rating using the funnel-down approach.

1. DEFINE each domain to understand how it's measured
2. Overall star rating and domain score – FACTS
3. Individual domains – FACTS
4. Each individual metric within each domain – FACTS
5. STOP and ask questions to create an action plan.

Step 1: use the DEFINE tool to understand how each individual domain is measured (Table 8.1). Keep in mind the star rating is a culmination of seven domains and 50+ metrics. Over time, the methodology may change, so review the CMS website to determine the current domains, metrics, and weights of each domain. As an example, the DEFINE tool using the mortality domain is as follows:

- Denominator: Medicare inpatient

- Exclusion criteria: varies by individual metric. Patients enrolled in Medicare for 12 months prior to hospitalization and left against medical advice
- Factor: risk-adjusted rate
- Inclusion criteria: *International Classification of Diseases* (ICD) codes vary by metric, Medicare inpatient
- Numerator: patient expirations within 30 days post hospitalization based on inclusion criteria
- Evaluate: mortality domain is a seven-metric measure that includes various disease groups utilizing a logistic regression model to risk-adjust the data.

After knowing your numbers using the DEFINE tool, step 2 in the funnel-down approach is to take a step back and focus on the FACTS of a hospital's star rating and individual domain scores utilizing a dashboard to graphically display the data (Figure 8.6). The FACTS are as follows:

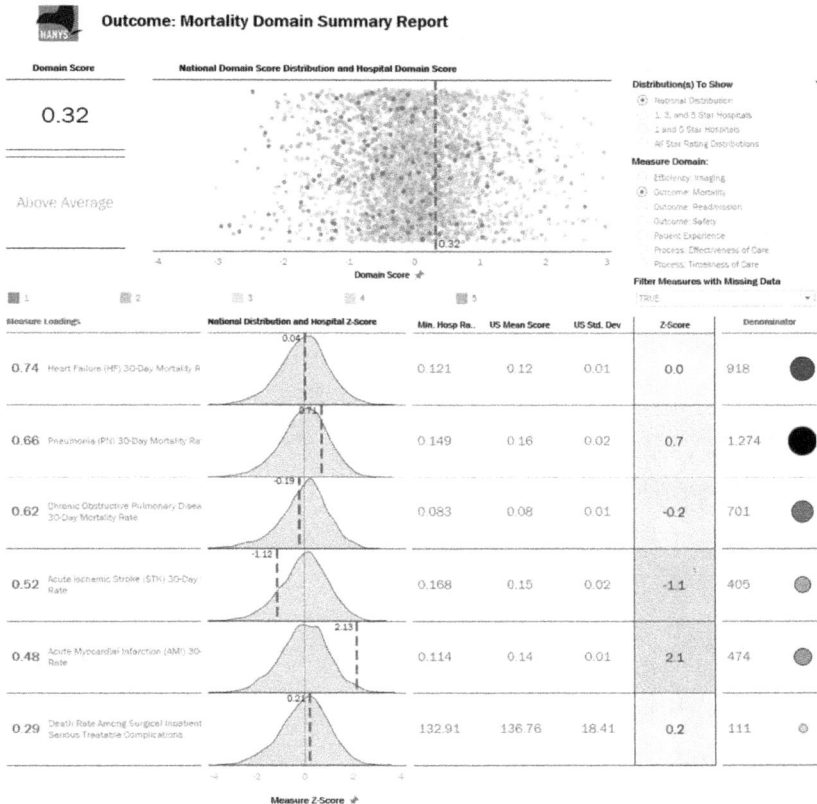

Figure 8.6 Healthcare Association of New York State (HANYS) Centers for Medicare/Medicaid Services (CMS) Star dashboard.

Source: Healthcare Association of New York State, 2017.

- Formulas: z-score, averages, standard deviation, confidence intervals, and percentiles
- Analyze patterns/trends: wide confidence intervals across domains indicate variability within measures
- Consider guidelines/rules: consider the proximity of the cutoff score for moving into a different star
- Think: domain weights vary, with highest-weighted domains having a bigger influence on the star rating. Do star rating metrics appear in other programs?
- Statistics: percentiles, domain scores, cutoff score, confidence intervals, domain, and hospital scores.

In Figure 8.7, Hospital A is a 3-star hospital with a final summary score or z-score of −0.29 with domain z-scores ranging from −1.770 to 2.270. Take note of the distribution range between −2.0 and 2.0 and where the cutoff points are for each star. Approximately, a 1-star hospital has a z-score below around −1.0, 2 stars is between −1.0 and −0.4, 3 stars between -0.4 and 0.2, 4 stars between 0.2 and 0.8, and 5 stars above 0.8. Comparing the individual domains to the cutoff scores in the distribution allows an additional interpretation of what star that domain would have. Readmission has a z-score of −1.770, which is equivalent to a 1-star rating and safety has a z-score of 2.270, which is in the 5-star rating. As a result, a 3-star hospital does not mean all domains are 3 stars. The advantage of a standard

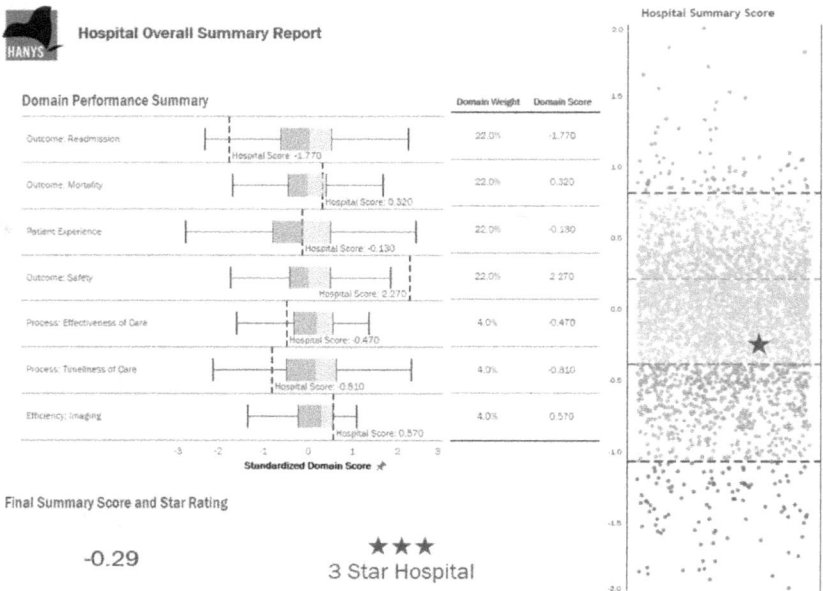

Figure 8.7 Centers for Medicare/Medicaid Services (CMS) Star Rating dashboard. Source: Healthcare Association of New York State, 2017.

normal distribution is that z–score ranges, population average, and population standard deviation are likely to be comparable to future releases. Theoretically, the knowledge of this distribution could be used to estimate a star rating for individual domains and individual metrics within the domain for future releases. The statistics may not be exact, but they would provide a frame of reference to understand how changes in metrics impact the star rating.

Knowing the box-and-whisker plot provides the 25th, 50th, and 75th percentile and a 99% confidence interval allows a quick comparison of a hospital's performance relative to the hospitals included in the analysis. Analyze a score falling within the box to determine if it falls in the 25th, 50th, or 75th percentile based on where the value is displayed. The middle line in the box represents the 50th percentile, the left side of the box represents the 25th percentile, and the right side of the box represents the 75th percentile. For example, the patient experience domain z–score of −0.130 is at the 50th percentile and mortality z–score 0.320 is close to the 75th percentile.

Moving on from the interpretation of the z–score, take into consideration the percentiles and width of the whiskers. A review of the whiskers on the plot shows the variability of performance within that domain. The advantage is to use this variability as knowledge for how the rest of the country is doing. Smaller boxes and whiskers indicate that hospitals have similar performance on that domain. Larger boxes and whiskers indicate inconsistency across hospitals for that domain. For example, the patient experience domain has the largest whiskers and the imaging domain has the shortest whiskers.

To further utilize the funnel-down approach from the overall hospital domain and star rating, step 3 focuses on individual domains along with their respective weights and domain scores. Take the time to DEFINE the individual domains to understand how each domain is measured along with the metrics that make up that domain. Focus on the FACTS in the graphical representation in Figure 8.6 with the box-and-whiskers plot and z–score.

The overall domain weights of the metrics show how much influence individual domains have on the overall z–score. For example, in Figure 8.6 the imaging domain has a z–score of 0.570, which is in the 75th percentile, but a weight of 4% means the influence on the overall star rating is less than other domains with a 22% weight. The implication is that a significant improvement in a domain score with a weight of 4% will impact the overall z–score less than a domain weighted 22%. Each of the individual metrics within a domain also influences the overall score for that domain. This influence on an overall domain can be seen by the **measure loading** in Figure 8.6 where scores close to 1 indicate a higher influence. This means that the heart failure (HF) 30-day mortality rate has a loading of 0.74, which is higher than the 0.29 for death rate among surgical inpatient serious treatable complications.

The question remains: where to focus? Domains with the highest weight? Measures with the highest loading? Or measures with the highest denominator? Domains closest to the next star level? And so on. This is a complicated discussion and warrants further review within your organization. In this example, we opted to focus on the mortality domain due to its high weight (22%) and ability to impact other governmental programs that include mortality metrics. The next step would be to determine which metric within the mortality domain to focus on. You may want to look at two metrics before deciding. Measures with the highest loading and highest denominator may be a place to start the conversation. The caveat is, what should you do when all measure loadings are high or what is considered a high measure loading? Is a 0.74 that much higher than a 0.66? The answer is that it may not be. This is why it's important to consider multiple metrics besides just the measure loading. One additional piece of information is the denominator. The HF mortality has a denominator of 918 and the pneumonia mortality rate has a denominator of 1,274. A larger denominator could indicate more opportunity for having an impact, but the pneumonia mortality has a z-score of 0.7, which puts it above the 50th percentile and the hospital mortality rate was 0.149 or 14.9%, which is lower than the US mean rate of 0.16 or 16.0%. It's not easy to decide where to improve, but a methodological approach can help.

Step 4 builds on the previous step to aid in further determining where to focus. At this phase in the funnel-down approach we move towards the detail of the metrics within each domain to narrow down a plan to focus improvement efforts. Continue utilizing the DEFINE tool to understand how measures are assessed and the FACTS tool to interpret the data. Similar to the discussion on control charts and the patient safety survey, high performance on a domain doesn't mean improvement is not warranted and low performance on a domain doesn't mean all metrics are low. It is possible for low domain scores to contain higher performance metrics and high domain scores to contain lower performance metrics. There is something learned from both exceptional and poor performance. For example, the safety domain (z-score = 2.270) resulted in performance equivalent to a 5-star rating, but the readmission domain (z-score = −1.770) was a 1-star rating. Does this mean we should ignore the safety domain and focus efforts on the readmission domain?

The advantage of methodological thinking is that the same approach is used for all analyses. The information used at the summary score level, domain level, or individual metric level is consistent. The FACTS don't change; rather the story becomes clearer on where to ACT.

- Formulas – standard deviation – n size in denominator, rates are risk-adjusted, z-scores are calculated using hospital average, population average and standard deviation.
- Analyze patterns/trends – national domain score distribution and hospital domain score distribution show that a 1-star hospital can have 5-star ratings and vice versa.
- Consider rules/guidelines – measure loadings close to 1 have a higher influence. Use z-score guidelines to interpret values
- Think – standard normal distribution; 68% of hospitals within 1 SD (z-score between −1 and 1), and 95% of hospitals within 2 SD. Measure loadings indicate the metrics that influence the domain score the most. Population average is large, so volume of data in future may have little impact on the population

average. Formulas for z-scores indicate the ability to calculate future z-scores with different data.

• Statistics – measure loadings, z-scores, average rates (population and hospital), population standard deviation, and volume.

All statistics tell different pieces of the same story. The FACTS of the individual metrics on Figure 8.6 identify measure loadings, hospital averages, population averages, population standard deviations, z-scores, and denominators. The factor loadings range from 0 to 1 and indicate the strength or influence an individual metric has on the overall domain score. A measure loading is similar in interpretation to the domain weight where values closer to 1 have a stronger influence on the overall domain score. The z-score and distribution show the nationwide distribution for a given metric along with how hospitals scored on that metric. Take note that the graphical distribution is similar to a bell-shaped curve, which is accomplished through a standard normal distribution of converting raw scores into z-scores. The hospital raw score corresponds to the conversion of the z-score into a raw score format. For example, a z-score of 0.04 for HF mortality corresponds to a 0.121 or 12.1% mortality rate. The US mean score and standard deviation provide a reference as to where a hospital rate compares to the US rate. The denominator provides the overall volume for each metric to better understand how many patients are used to calculate that metric.

Taking a step back and focusing on the statistics displayed serves as a methodological approach to analyzing data and determining where to focus improvement efforts. All hospitals continually improve, so the 5-star rating continues to be a moving target. Capitalize on what a hospital does well and continually refine processes. Be the one others try to beat! Figure 8.6 is the mortality domain that this hospital is performing above average on. Look at the pneumonia mortality metric. The z-score is 0.71, which is equivalent to a 0.149 or 14.9% mortality rate. The US rate is 0.16 or 16%, with a standard deviation of 0.02 or 2%. The measure loading is 0.66 and the denominator is 1,274, which indicates a high volume metric with a high influence on the overall domain.

Before thinking that a high measure loading with a high volume (denominator) is the best place to focus efforts to improve, let's take it one step further and simulate a scenario through leveraging statistics. The z-score formula requires the hospital average, population average, and population standard deviation. Considering the denominator is provided means it is possible to calculate the numerator. For example, a 14.9% pneumonia mortality rate with a denominator of 1,274 means the numerator is 189.8 or rounded to 190 (0.149 × 1,274). Knowing the population average and standard deviation may not change too much and assuming the new hospital denominator stays relatively consistent, it is possible to simulate changes in z-scores with new data. What would a new z-score be if mortalities increase by 10, which increases the numerator from 190 to 200? Assuming the denominator remains the same at 1,274, the new mortality rate would be 15.7% (200/1,274). Converting the new mortality rate (15.7%) into a z-score using the population average (16%) and population standard deviation (2%) results in a new z-score of 0.2. In referring to Figure 8.6, the original 0.7 z-score is a 4-star rating and the new 0.2 z-score could be either a 3- or low 4-star rating. The moral of the story is that small changes can result in change. Minimal changes like 10 additional mortalities on a high-performing metric could change the outcome to a low-performing metric.

A caveat to the calculations is how precise the statistics are. Rounding to the nearest value potentially impacts the overall calculations. For example, if a mortality rate of 13% is rounded to the nearest percentage, then the rate has the possibility of ranging between 12.5% and 13.4% and still equals 13%. The same applies to a 12% population average, which could range between 11.5% and 12.4%, and a 1% population standard deviation could range from 0.5% to 1.4%. Tables 8.3–8.6 simulate the impact statistical precision has on overall z-scores. Negative z-scores imply that the hospital average is worse than the population average and positive z-scores indicate hospital average is lower than population average.

Tables 8.3–8.6 portray a variety of scenarios that impact the precision of statistics. The first three data points in Table 8.3 all have a difference of 1% between the hospital and population average with varying standard deviations resulting in a z-score between −0.71 and −2.00. The last two data points examine two scenarios with the maximum standard deviation (1.4%). One simulates the lowest (12.5%) hospital average compared to the highest (12.4%) population average and the other simulates the highest (13.4%) hospital with the lowest (11.5%) population average. The result is a z-score of −0.07 and −1.36, respectively. The conclusion is a 1% difference in averages with a smaller standard deviation results in a high z-score and a 1% difference in average with a larger standard deviation results in a z-score closer to 0 in this scenario. Three other scenarios are simulated with varying population averages, hospital averages, and population standard deviations. Table 8.4 examines the impact of a z-score with varying population averages and results in z-scores ranging from −0.60 to −1.50. Table 8.5 measures the impact on a varying hospital average with a z-score ranging between −0.50 and −1.40. Table 8.6 examines the variability in standard deviation and results in z-scores ranging between −0.71 and −2.0. The general conclusion is that the more precise the statistical estimates are, the more accurate the calculation would be. To put it into perspective, a −2.0 z-score is a 1-star rating, a 0.20–0.8 z-score is a 4-star rating, and above a 0.8 z-score is a 5-star rating.

Step 5 is to STOP and ask questions to develop an action plan. As the country continues to advance, the quest to 5 stars is a continually moving target. A critical review of the analysis with a methodological approach demonstrates the beneficial aspects of utilizing multiple statistics to tell a story and not jump to conclusions about being a 3-star hospital. While the desire may be a 5-star hospital, this is a great long-term, but maybe not so realistic, goal. Focusing on the FACTS identified patterns/trends in data that showcase a 3-star hospital has the potential for individual metrics to be at a 5- or 1-star rating. The action plan moving forward provides a plan to capitalize on this knowledge to hit those moving targets. Continuing with the mortality domain, the STOP action plan could be as follows:

Table 8.3 Impact of z-scores with varying averages and standard deviation

Hospital average	Population average	Population standard deviation	z-score
12.5%	11.5%	0.5%	−2.00
13.0%	12.0%	1.0%	−1.00
13.4%	12.4%	1.4%	−0.71
12.5%	12.4%	1.4%	−0.07
13.4%	11.5%	1.4%	−1.36

Table 8.4 Impact of z-scores with varying population average

Hospital average	Population average	Population standard deviation	z-score
13.0%	11.5%	1.0%	−1.50
13.0%	12.0%	1.0%	−1.00
13.0%	12.4%	1.0%	−0.60

Table 8.5 Impact of z-scores with varying hospital average

Hospital average	Population average	Population standard deviation	z-score
12.5%	12.0%	1.0%	−0.50
13.0%	12.0%	1.0%	−1.00
13.4%	12.0%	1.0%	−1.40

Table 8.6 Impact of z-scores with varying population standard deviation

Hospital average	Population average	Population standard deviation	z-score
13.0%	12.0%	0.5%	−2.00
13.0%	12.0%	1.0%	−1.00
13.0%	12.0%	1.4%	−0.71

- SMART goal – improve the mortality domain score by decreasing the pneumonia morality rate by 10% over the next year.
- Think critically – a 10% reduction would be decreasing the acute pneumonia mortality rate from 14.9% to 13.4%. Assuming the denominator is consistent, how many patients would need to be reduced from the numerator to achieve a 10% reduction? AMI z-score is 2.1, which rates in the 5-star category. What processes are working well for AMI that may apply to pneumonia, if possible? Does pneumonia mortality appear in financial initiatives?
- Operationalization of your metrics – the mortality rate on the star rating is risk-adjusted using a logistic regression model with populations defined by specific diagnosis codes.

- Purpose – calculate the 3-year average raw rate for pneumonia to compare that with the CMS Star Rating rate. This will provide a relative idea of what the raw rate is compared to the risk-adjusted rate (the z-score converted into a raw score). Develop a process map for pneumonia to determine metrics to trend. Examine process metrics for metric z-scores that are above average and determine if processes apply to pneumonia.

Discussion

A common theme from previous chapters was implementing initiatives towards changing behavior to impact outcomes. Any intervention requiring human interaction is subject to resistance. Overcoming these barriers and implementing successful change begin with the right tools. Remember, the best predictor of future performance is past behavior (Wernimont & Campbell, 1968). The CMS Star Rating provides data from the past with varying timeframes included in the analysis. While the data may not be as concurrent as desired to take action, organizations cannot control the public's perception of these ratings, nor change the outcome. As a result, discounting the 3 years of data as being old doesn't change the outcome for three reasons: (1) the star rating will still be released; (2) the next release includes two of those 3 years; and (3) any change implemented today will take a year or two to be included in the performance period and will be included in the next few releases.

A wealth of information exists beyond the four walls of a healthcare organization. Capitalize on the availability of various metrics to serve as benchmarks and create a story from available statistics. The CMS Star Rating provides data from healthcare organizations that is vital to not only compete to be a 5-star organization, but shed light into how other organizations are performing. In order to be the best, you need to know and beat the best. This is done through reflecting on data and maximizing the story to drive future improvements. Utilize current data within your organization to trend what is happening now to better understand what the impact may be when the new performance period for the star rating comes around.

While it's not possible to change the past, focus improvement efforts on the present to change the future. You can't change what happened, you likely can't change what is happening, but you can change what will happen. Every door presents an opportunity with two outcomes: being reactive or proactive. Don't wait for the change; be the change. The choice begins with you and you can continue to react and deflect or face the facts through proactive improvement to change the future. The CMS Star Rating serves as a tool for evaluating historical performance to determine where to focus improvement efforts and compare your performance to others. Many types of statistics aid in the interpretation and development of meaningful stories. Take a step back and review the available statistics. With a little creativity and insight into various statistical formulas, leverage this knowledge to estimate the future impact of what will happen. Know that you cannot solve every problem, so rely on others for support and guidance. Inquiring with others is an effective way to incorporate alternative perspectives for a complete picture of what is happening. Don't set goals for the sake of setting goals. STOP and develop a plan to hit those moving targets.

Success isn't easy and failure is likely, but persistence and dedication sustain through the failures. If at first you don't succeed, fix the process and reach for the stars. It only takes one person to initiate change, but a team to implement and sustain change. Be the innovator by leveraging the statistics and methodology of the CMS Star data to drive future behavioral initiatives towards hitting those moving targets on the path to a 5-star hospital.

Discussion Questions

- How do publicly reported metrics alter your perspective of initiating change in your organization?
- How does the CMS Star Rating impact your decision making?
- When developing initiatives in your organization, what value do you see in focusing not only on the outcome, but the processes as well?
- What are your thoughts on these two statements: (1) fixing a problem not fully understood will not result in improvement; and (2) fixing an outcome metric without understanding the process will not result in improvement?
- When faced with making improvement decisions, using the CMS Star Rating where would you focus first? 1-star or 5-star domains? Did the discussed approach change your perspective?

9   CMS Hospital Compare

"Analyzing data begins and ends with STATISTICS. You cannot ACT without the FACTS."

Introduction

Knowledge is power and data is used to drive knowledge, power, and decisions. Decisions are made daily based on FACTS, beliefs, hunches, or previous data. So why do some decisions result in sustainable change and others don't? Is it better to utilize previous experience and beliefs as opposed to the facts that data provides? Some may argue that personal experience may be more effective, because numbers lie. Others may say that personal experience is biased, so numbers are more effective. Regardless of your personal stance, the amount of available data in healthcare continues to grow exponentially. Being able to critically evaluate statistics is an effective tool to understand whether the people or the numbers are lying.

A well-known book entitled *How to Lie with Statistics* by Huff and Geis was originally published in 1954 and reissued in 1993. It depicts the story of errors inferred from interpreting statistics (Huff, 1993). These errors may be a result of human interpretation (i.e., people lie) or graphical depiction of the numbers (i.e., statistics lie). While a graphical representation of statistics or multiple types of statistics tell different stories, being able to critically evaluate all statistics helps overcome the potential "lies." Hunches, beliefs, or gut feelings will only go so far. A training program titled *More Than a Gut Feeling* has multiple versions and focuses on the premise of not relying on a gut feeling when interviewing applicants. Moreover, hunches, beliefs, and gut feelings have the potential to lead to assumptions. Assumptions are confirmed through experience that may lead to the appearance of facts, when in reality all that's left is a story with the appearance of facts based on the culmination of experience and assumptions. Consider the following short passage on assumptions.

This is a story about four people named Everybody, Somebody, Anybody and Nobody. There was an important job to be done and Everybody was sure that Somebody would do it. Anybody could have done it, but Nobody did it. Somebody got angry about that, because it was Everybody's job. Everybody thought Anybody could do it, but Nobody realized that Everybody wouldn't do it. It ended up that Everybody blamed Somebody when Nobody did what Anybody could have.

(Naylor & Ricco, 2013)

This simple reflection on making decisions and achieving results demonstrates the importance of never losing focus on the story told by the results. Step back and don't jump to conclusions by making sure all information is collected prior to deriving conclusions. The FACTS ensure no assumptions or gut feelings are used by forcing methodological critical thinking to analyze data.

The previous chapters provided a variety of statistics, programs, and initiatives revolving around healthcare and metrics used to drive decision making and performance. Interpreting statistics is challenging, but the right tools make the process of drawing conclusions easier. These tools and processes take advantage of available data prior to making decisions. This final analytic chapter focuses on a combination of data presented earlier (i.e., Hospital Compare: www.medicare.gov/hospitalcompare/ and https://data.medicare.gov), and these are resources for analyzing metrics impacting the Medicare population.

Upon reviewing the Hospital Compare website, one piece of information available is planning ahead. Patients are becoming more analytically savvy with expectations about care delivery and positive outcomes are increasing. When patients have the luxury of planning ahead, then educated decisions using publicly available data is a place to start. The reputation of Centers for Medicare/Medicaid Services (CMS) and the validity of their data make using the CMS website a place for patients to start analyzing data to make healthcare decisions. Hospital Compare provides a guide to choosing a hospital (www.medicare.gov/Pubs/pdf/10181.pdf). Healthcare is transforming from a place to receive care to a customer-oriented place where patients *choose* to go. This "choice" may not be made on a hunch, belief, or gut feeling that the outcome will be positive, but rather by examining actual facts. The drive to better understand health information stems from a lack of satisfaction with information provided by clinicians and a desire to expand options for diagnosis/treatment, and to be better informed (i.e., determining questions in advance) during their appointment (Kivits, 2006). Reasons for being more informed should not be viewed as a bad thing, but rather patients taking responsibility for their health. Patients are making informed decisions on where to receive care based on outcomes. Hospital Compare provides information on Medicare patients only, but not all patients receiving hospital care are Medicare patients. Patients may generalize results (external validity) from the Medicare population to their own personal situation or they may not even think about the fact or know that these results are based on Medicare patients.

As discussed in Chapter 1, many internet sites provide data on various comparisons of patient populations and outcomes. While the validity of these websites is questionable, Hospital Compare data comes from CMS and is the same data utilized for financial/performance penalties/incentives in some of the initiatives discussed in Chapter 7 as well as the CMS Star Rating. Although data from Hospital Compare is delayed, and some patients may not look at the details of what data is displayed, the moral of the story is that the best defense is a great offense. Being reactive to the results presented doesn't fix the problem. Being pro-active and knowing your numbers to create change lead to meaningful conclusions and interventions impacting care.

That being said, focusing on the FACTS when analyzing data is key to deriving these meaningful conclusions. Any decision made without facts won't fix the situation. Dissect the data, sources, and statistics to understand the implications made as a result of the data presented. Data is all around and with the enhancing of technology the availability of data will grow exponentially, making those targets move at a rapid pace. Data can be quantitative or qualitative and comes from statistics publicly reported (i.e., Hospital Compare), magazines, CMS, patient experience, Agency for Healthcare Research and Quality (AHRQ), Joint Commission, Dartmouth Atlas, radio/TV advertisements, billboards, professional journals, personal patient experiences, and so on. Any of the aforementioned data sources has the potential to influence patients' future healthcare decisions regarding where he/she *chooses* to receive care.

Methodology

Understanding statistics begins with the methodology of how data is calculated and where data originates from. Hospital Compare provides a wealth of information on hospitals:

- General information – pertains to basic demographic information (i.e., name, address, phone number, type of hospital, etc.) about a hospital.
- Patient experience – data from individual patient experience items. Refer to Chapter 5.
- Timely and effective care – process metrics related to various disease conditions.
- Complications – outcome metrics as a result of certain surgical procedures.
- Readmissions and deaths – risk-adjusted rates comparing performance on various disease conditions compared to national rates. See Chapter 4 on interpreting mortality and readmissions.
- Use of medical imaging – process metrics related to outpatient medical imaging.
- Payment and value of care – financial comparisons of hospital performance on patient outcomes compared to the national average.

The above categories of metrics correspond to over 100 different types of metrics currently available within Hospital Compare. These metrics are inclusive of the more than 50 metrics included in the star rating. Details on all of the metrics are found on Hospital Compare (www.medicare.gov/hospitalcompare/Data/Data-Updated.html#). Considering definitions and metrics change over time, it's critically important to review Hospital Compare for the latest data definitions and most up-to-date information.

The methodology portion is broken into two sections. The first section is the methodology of data definitions and the second section is the methodology of statistical analyses. An example using two categories (complications and readmissions and deaths) is included.

Methodology of Data Definitions

Making data-based decisions requires an understanding of how metrics are operationalized. The complications category of measures contains two distinct types of metrics. The first is surgical complications and the second is healthcare-associated infections. Within the realm of surgical complications, there are 11 different metrics available. An argument could be made that there are more than 11 considering one complication metric is a composite (PSI-90, which is an aggregated measure of multiple other metrics). There are six healthcare-associated infection metrics available. As for the readmission and death category, this is broken into readmissions, containing eight metrics, and mortality, containing six metrics.

To keep this chapter concise, the DEFINE tool is applied to one metric from each category. HAI-2 (catheter-associated urinary tract infections (CAUTI) in intensive care units (ICUs) and select non-ICUs) was chosen from the healthcare-associated infection (HAI) metric. The readmission and death metric chosen from the deaths is MORT-30-PN (pneumonia 30-day mortality rate) (Table 9.1).

Table 9.1 DEFINE tool examples

DEFINE tool	HAI-2	MORT-30-PN
Denominator	All inpatient hospital patients in an ICU, medical, surgical, or medical/surgical unit	All patients with index admission of pneumonia
Exclusion criteria	Patients with a catheter in place less than 2 days or no clinical indicators for infection	Enrolled in Medicare 12 months prior to hospitalization, transfers from another acute care facility, left AMA, inconsistent data
Factor	Standardized infection ratio (SIR) – calculation is observed number of infections divided by expected number of infections	Risk-adjusted mortality rate – calculation is risk-adjusted based on age, past medical history, and comorbidities
Inclusion criteria	All patients with a catheter in place for more than 2 days and meeting clinical criteria for infection	Medicare patients 65 or older with principal or secondary ICD diagnosis codes
Numerator	Number of infections	Number of deaths within 30 days post discharge
Evaluate	Metric is a SIR, which is risk-adjusted from NHSN. Data is updated quarterly and contains a year of data	Metric is risk-adjusted based on Medicare claims data. Data is updated annually and contains 3 years of data

AMA, against medical advice; HAI-2, healthcare-associated infections 2; ICD, *International Classification of Diseases;* ICU, intensive care unit; MORT-30-PN, pneumonia 30-day mortality rate; NHSN, National Healthcare Safety Network.

The story derived from utilizing the DEFINE tool provides a complete picture of how metrics are operationalized. Using these two measures as examples, it's important to note the general theme is that data provided on Hospital Compare is risk-adjusted. Replicating this with an individual hospital's data is not possible because the statistics regarding the model development are not provided. As a result, it is not possible to replicate this exact data using a hospital's own data. However, arguments regarding the timeliness of data availability have led some organizations to utilize the inclusion/exclusion criteria to monitor performance more concurrently, with the caveat that it will not be the same as CMS. This applies more to mortality and readmission data as the 3 years of data analyzed on Hospital Compare can contain data from, at most, 5 years ago, from the most current year up to 2 years from the current year. Understanding the implications for improvement on data from 2 years ago poses challenges. The data analyzed is a rolling 3 years, so 1 year of data is included in the same analysis three times. For example, if the current timeframe of data available is July 2016–June 2019, then the next release year will include July 2017–June 2020, and the third release will be July 2018–June 2021. As you can see, the year 2019 is included in all three releases.

Methodology of Statistics

Knowing the operationalization of metrics (i.e., construct validity) is one piece to the analytic puzzle. The other piece is to understand the various statistics presented and how to leverage them to make decisions or tell an effective objective story. Hospital Compare provides over 100 metrics, with the most common statistics being risk-adjusted metrics, confidence intervals, and statistical significance. For purposes of consistency, the HAI complications and readmission/death categories are used as examples.

Within the complications category, the statistics include rates, ratios, and a composite metric. Don't assume the rates included in complications are multiplied by 100 because this may not be true. Don't assume that a ratio is a comparison between values either. The PSI-3 (pressure ulcer rate) is an observed rate multiplied by 1,000. The advice in Chapter 3 was to focus on the words preceding the word "ratio." HAI-2 (CAUTI) is a standardized infection ratio (SIR), which means the ratio in this definition is risk-adjusted. The moral of the story is that understanding and analyzing data take time. Jumping to conclusions leads to erroneous assumptions about what stories the data is telling, so take the time to DEFINE.

The next statistical concept presented within Hospital Compare is confidence intervals. Confidence intervals are useful in understanding what a hospital's population metric would be given a sample of data. For example, the pneumonia mortality rate is a risk-adjusted metric based on Medicare patients. Other metrics within Hospital Compare provide data on Medicare patients, so it's important to have a way to reflect the entire population as hospitals treat non-Medicare patients. The confidence interval allows you to estimate what, in this case, your pneumonia mortality rate would be for the entire hospital.

To begin with the confidence interval surrounding the SIR, Hospital Compare utilizes the National Healthcare Safety Network (NHSN) for infection data. The SIR is calculated using a logistic regression modeling technique where model estimates are calculated at the 95% confidence interval. With respect to mortality/readmission, Hospital Compare analyzes data on Medicare patients aged 65 and older. There are wo plausible explanations for the use of a confidence interval:

1. The mortality and readmission rates provided are risk-adjusted and may not be the actual hospital rate, so the logistic regression model provides an estimate for the rate.
2. Hospitals do not only serve Medicare patients, so the risk-adjusted rates are based on the Medicare population and not the hospital population.

As we have mentioned, the main purpose of the confidence interval is to state with confidence that the population rate will fall within the calculated interval. The next question revolves around the interpretation of the confidence interval and how to implement it in practice. The task of interpreting the confidence interval starts with how the information is presented. Hospital Compare draws conclusions using confidence intervals based on statistical significance using three different interpretations: (1) better than national rate; (2) no different than national rate; (3) worse than national rate. The statistical significance and conclusions derived from the presented results vary based on the metric being analyzed.

For the purpose of HAI complications, the SIR, with its respective 95% confidence interval, is compared to the benchmark of 1.0. A value above 1.0 indicates that performance is worse than expected and a value below 1.0 indicates that performance is better than expected. The statistical significance is interpreted one of three ways based on the confidence interval containing 1.0. If the confidence interval contains 1.0, then the hospital is determined to be no different than the

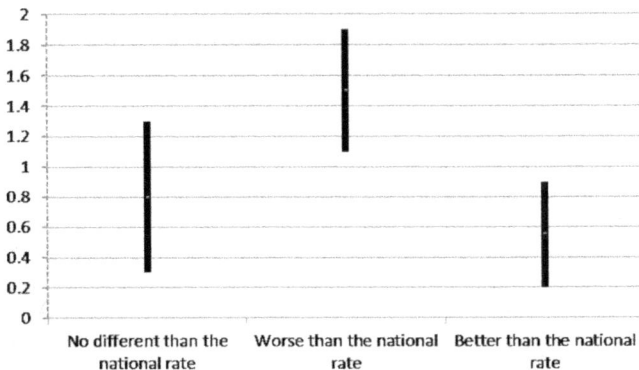

Figure 9.1 Confidence intervals depicting statistical significance.

national rate. If 1.0 is not included in the confidence interval, then to determine whether the hospital performance is better or worse is based on reviewing the entire confidence interval as being above or below 1.0. When the confidence interval is above 1.0, this indicates worse than the national rate and below 1.0 indicates better than the national rate (see Figure 9.1 for a visual display of confidence intervals).

A similar interpretation for readmission and death metrics is used to determine statistical significance. The only slight variation is that the interpretation is not based on 1.0, but rather the national rate calculated by CMS. This means the national rate may vary by metric. The remaining interpretation is the same. If the confidence interval for the risk-adjusted mortality/readmission rate contains the national rate, then the interpretation is no different than the national rate. Performing significantly better than the national rate requires the entire confidence interval to be below the national rate and performing worse than the national rate requires the entire confidence interval to be above the national rate.

Results

Methodologically understanding the process that results in the calculation of the statistics, and how the metric is defined, is critical to being able to use the results to tell a story. For the analysis of the mortality rate from Hospital Compare, the same three steps are used: (1) DEFINE the metric; (2) focus on the FACTS of what is presented; (3) STOP and ask questions to plan for improvement. A methodological approach to analyzing data and spending time inquiring what others are doing to gather all available data before drawing conclusions is the key to success. Visually displaying statistics to effectively tell the story is challenging. The end result of any visual display should drive more questions than answers. As with previous chapters, there are many ways to present data effectively and Figure 9.2

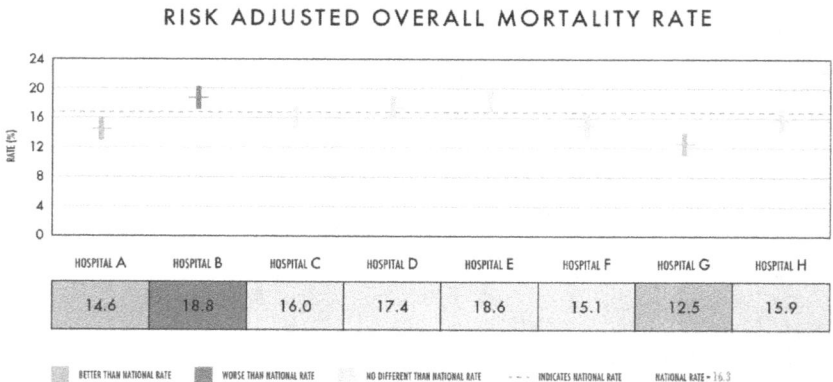

RISK ADJUSTED OVERALL MORTALITY RATE

HOSPITAL A	HOSPITAL B	HOSPITAL C	HOSPITAL D	HOSPITAL E	HOSPITAL F	HOSPITAL G	HOSPITAL H
14.6	18.8	16.0	17.4	18.6	15.1	12.5	15.9

BETTER THAN NATIONAL RATE   WORSE THAN NATIONAL RATE   NO DIFFERENT THAN NATIONAL RATE   - - - INDICATES NATIONAL RATE   NATIONAL RATE = 16.3

Figure 9.2 Funnel-down approach: the big picture.

is one potential display of data. Continuing with the trend of the funnel-down approach to analyzing data, the big picture starts at the top of the funnel.

DEFINE the Metric

Prior to the analysis of any statistics, a methodological approach to understanding how the metric is defined ensures the right actions are taken. This approach forces you to step back and not jump to conclusions about what interventions initiate improvement. Using the DEFINE tool for the risk-adjusted overall mortality rate yields:

- Denominator – all discharged Medicare patients over 65 years old
- Exclusion criteria – patients enrolled into Medicare hospital program on day 1 of admission and enrollment 12 months prior to admission, patients leaving against medical advice (AMA)
- Factor – risk-adjusted rate using a logistic regression model. Patients with multiple admissions in a year have one randomly chosen for inclusion in the model
- Inclusion criteria – Medicare patients over 65 years old. No disease-specific selection, so all diagnoses
- Numerator – all deaths within 30 days of discharge
- Evaluate – the mortality rate is a risk-adjusted rate using all Medicare patients over the age of 65. The rate provided on CMS Hospital Compare is a rolling 3-year average that is updated throughout the year. Mortalities within 30 days post hospitalization are included in the numerator.

The DEFINE tool indicates that the rate being analyzed is a 3-year risk-adjusted trend of all Medicare patients over the age of 65. There are minor exclusions based on enrollment in a hospice program, patients who left AMA for specific conditions (acute myocardial infarction and heart failure), and other exclusions based on the disease condition being analyzed. Additionally, mortalities occurring within 30 days after leaving the hospital do count towards the hospital's mortality rate. Every analyzed metric benefits from the DEFINE tool to understand nuances between metrics.

Focus on the FACTS of What Is Presented

All analyses begin and end with statistics. This is why the FACTS tool begins with formulas and ends with statistics. It is difficult to ACT on data without statistics. Once metrics are fully understood, the next step is to focus on the FACTS. Assumptions made from presented data without thoroughly understanding the statistics displayed on the graph are ineffective.

- Formulas:
    - 95% confidence interval: indicates data was collected based on a sample of patients and the interval provided is a reflection of what the actual

hospital rate could be for all patients. The sample size impacts the width of the confidence interval. A smaller sample results in a larger confidence interval and a larger sample results in a smaller confidence interval.

- National and hospital rate: risk-adjusted average rate.

- Analyze patterns/trends – 3 years of trended data displayed using confidence intervals. Rates allow for a quick comparison of hospitals that may be performing better or worse than the national rate. Hospitals A, F, and H may have similar rates, but one is performing better. Hospital E has a larger confidence interval, but a similar rate to Hospital B. Hospital B is performing worse than the national rate.

- Consider guidelines/rules – statistical significance for confidence intervals is based on whether or not the entire confidence interval is above or below the national rate.

- Think – a visual display provides a lot of information. There are clear differences in performance from a statistical perspective. What are Hospitals A and G doing that is different from Hospital B? Do Hospitals A and G have a higher volume since the confidence intervals are smaller? How can Hospitals C, F, and H, which all have a lower rate than the national rate, become statistically better than the nation?

- Statistics – confidence interval, risk-adjusted rate, national rate, and statistical significance.

Focusing on the FACTS provides a structured way to think and interpret data prior to telling a story. Considering a picture is worth a thousand words, a key to avoiding assumptions/hunches/beliefs is remaining objective. Graphical visualizations can generate multiple interpretations, but a goal is to create a visual resulting in the same interpretation regardless of who looks at it.

Focusing on the FACTS shows the data presented is risk-adjusted with a confidence interval and a national rate as a benchmark. Testing your creativity and using insight to ask questions utilize knowledge to understand the hidden meaning behind statistics. For example, like standard deviation, the size of the confidence interval is a reflection of sample size. Hospitals with a small sample have a larger confidence interval (i.e., Hospital F) and a larger sample results in a smaller confidence interval (i.e., Hospitals A and G). This allows for finding the insight in variations on volume within that hospital. Hospital F has a lower volume of patients compared to Hospital A.

The last piece of the story is statistical significance. Hospital Compare provides information regarding statistical significance that implies a hospital with a confidence interval completely below the national rate (i.e., Hospitals A and G) is statistically performing better than the national rate. A hospital with a confidence interval completely above the national rate (i.e., Hospital B) is statistically performing worse than the national rate. Any hospital touching the national rate indicates no difference between the national rate. Questions may be different considering Hospital D has an average rate above the national rate and Hospital F has an average rate below the national rate, but both hospitals are performing no different.

STOP and Ask Questions to Plan for Improvement

The final step to storytelling with data is to leverage the methodological approach and statistical interpretation to develop behavioral-based interventions or process improvements for the future. Analyzing all available information is paramount to deriving conclusions from the statistics being presented. A proper plan can prevent poor performance. Having a plan for implementing an intervention begins with a plan, so STOP and ask questions.

- SMART goal – develop disease-specific interventions to reduce the current observed mortality rate by 5% in 1 year.
- Think critically – 3 years of historical data on Medicare patients over 65 years old. Confidence interval uses the model to provide estimates of the hospital's performance.
- Operationalize your metrics – displayed metric utilizes Medicare patients. Care doesn't change based on patient type. Leverage the knowledge of this metric and use the confidence interval as an estimate for the entire hospital population.
- Purpose – CMS Hospital Compare is a rolling 3-year rate. Any intervention put into place won't be reflective on Hospital Compare until a year or two later. Based on the goal, the approach could be to implement an intervention and determine process metrics to reduce the mortality rate now.

Chances are data drives more questions than answers. One question from these results is based on the data being a 3-year aggregate and may be considered old, because the next data release will likely include a year of data that's already passed. A hospital may have a year or more recent data than what is available on Hospital Compare, so current initiatives may take a year or two to be included in the analysis. As a result, impacting performance on a metric using data that's already passed or not being able to evaluate performance until a year or two later poses challenges. It's not possible to wait 2 years to see if an intervention is working, so why should I be concerned with this data? The short answer is these metrics may carry financial/performance incentives and/or penalties, so ignoring them is not an option.

Another challenge is Hospital Compare data is a risk-adjusted 30-day post-discharge mortality. Hospitals may only have access to in-hospital mortality, so they may not have the 30-day post-discharge data to determine whether or not a patient has passed away. As a result, an internal metric may not be a 100% accurate reflection of what is on the Hospital Compare website. This could create some concerns with how to impact a rate you can't calculate with data that's not readily available post hospitalization. Despite this other criticism, this data will still be included on financial/performance incentives/penalties. Internal data can serve as a potential estimate and a more concurrent option to monitor trends and small tests of change.

Discussion

The above criticisms – old data and unavailable data post hospitalization – are two of many potential barriers you may face when trying to use data to drive future improvement efforts.

The first criticism made regarding the data as old and not reflecting current performance may be true; this doesn't avoid the fact that every year of data is included in two future updates. Failure to address an issue could result in penalties over multiple years. The focus of improvement must remain on the patient and not critiquing the applicability of data from the past. Patients looking at Hospital Compare may not be interested in or pay close attention to the timeframe of when data is collected. The data is presented as rates and overall statistical significance, so finding the data collection time period and definitions requires additional clicks. Think about it for a minute. Do you believe a patient cares that the mortality rate provided is a 30-day post-hospital discharge rate or if it's an in-hospital mortality rate or understands the difference between a raw rate versus a risk-adjusted rate? Is it possible that a patient may view the mortality rate and wonder whether or not they will die as a result of receiving care at your hospital and not think about if they will die within 30 days of leaving the hospital? While a hospital may criticize the validity of the data, this doesn't stop patients from interpreting the results and choosing care based on the data they research. It's important to transition from defense to offense and move from reactive to proactive.

Drawing conclusions from statistics takes time and patience. Jumping to conclusions is never the right approach to interpreting data as assumptions, beliefs, and previous experience may take over, resulting in confirming your thoughts as opposed to understanding the story and the facts. Take the time to think methodologically prior to analyzing data. The DEFINE, FACTS, and STOP tools all utilize a methodological approach to statistical analyses and stimulate critical thinking. As the amount of data grows exponentially, you will be tested with creatively analyzing data in new ways using complex statistics that may be unfamiliar to you. A methodological approach allows you to break apart the metrics into meaningful pieces. Leveraging data drives many aspects of improvement and performance, such as making financial decisions, patient treatment decisions, and hospital performance decisions, as well as patients using data to make decisions on where to receive care. Data also has financial and performance implications.

Determining the most effective story to tell is never based on one statistic alone. Statistics, individually, provide one side of a story. Combining all statistics provides a more robust story and has more credibility through reducing alternative explanations. For example, if you only presented a raw mortality rate, then you open up the opportunity for someone to say patients at this hospital are sicker than others. If you include both the raw mortality rate and risk-adjusted mortality rate, then this question is resolved because the risk adjustment factors in variables influencing mortality. It won't stop the statement that "our patients are sicker," but it gives you a proactive response to the statement with statistics and facts using risk-adjusted metrics.

We need to move beyond the one story using one statistic and integrate various statistics together to tell a more effective story. Similarly, to elaborate on what was mentioned above, imagine if the only statistic provided was a 12% mortality rate. How would others know this is risk-adjusted or that it is a 30-day post-discharge mortality rate or that it is a raw mortality rate? How would it be possible to compare this rate to a benchmark? Simply stating a mortality rate is 12% is a fact. It may be one fact, but that doesn't provide much direction. Combining the mortality rate with a confidence interval and a national benchmark provides more information that leads to more critical questions. Likewise, combining multiple metrics together provides a bigger picture of the story. An ineffective story results in a one-word answer. An effective story generates enthusiasm and questions.

Interpreting statistics requires time, knowledge, and thinking. Not everyone has the luxury of time, knowledge, and thinking. A few simple tools built utilizing everyday language serve as a subliminal message to have that split second of a light bulb going off. This is the purpose of developing tools tied to language heard on a regular basis. DEFINE your metrics, focus on the FACTS, and STOP to ask questions are key phrases used to prime you to focus on a systematic approach to interpreting statistics. The message for each of the previous chapters is to focus on a methodological approach to analyzing data, setting goals to drive change, and ensuring the developed interventions are grounded in behavior, which are all key components to implement change. This chapter concludes the analysis of data using various initiatives/programs within healthcare. The final chapter is a culmination of the methodological approach to utilize the STATISTICS toolkit for storytelling with data.

Discussion Questions

- Think of situations where change was implemented based on experience and another situation where it was based on facts. What were the successes and failures of both approaches?
- Have you ever sat in a presentation where data was presented based on assumptions and experience, but the discussion was led to be fact? What were your reactions?
- Do you believe that patients are becoming more analytically savvy when making healthcare decisions? How can we as healthcare professionals assist in the decision making?
- How do external data sources (magazines, radio/TV advertisements, billboards, personal experience) shape your views on implementing change in healthcare? Do these same sources impact patients in the same way?
- How does data that is delayed by up to 2–5 years impact your decision making? Will patients react in the same way that you do? Would patients care that data presented on important health outcomes is 2 years old? If not, then why do we focus on that delay?

- How can you use confidence intervals to drive change? Would you approach change differently using confidence intervals where the average is below a national rate, but the confidence interval crosses the national rate or if the average rate is above the national rate, but the confidence interval crosses the national rate?

10 Turn Data Into Action

"Failure and mistakes are just reminders that you haven't found the right path to success."

Introduction

Statistics are all around us, whether you can see them or not. Throughout this entire book, the focus has been on critically evaluating data to understand what happened to make changes in the future. We can use data to create sustainable solutions that improve the actions of others or to leverage data to make more informed decisions (i.e., developing goals and improving patient outcomes). While it's important to focus on using data to drive innovative solutions, sometimes the change needs to come from within. Data can also be used to empower your own professional development. We are only as strong as our biggest weakness. While we may, at times, get wrapped up in the world around us and determine the best option for improving patient outcomes, we may focus less on improving ourselves. Leveraging the skills learned to ask questions and improve outcomes promotes critical thinking skills to apply in any situation. Throughout the previous chapters, the focus was on promoting critical thinking about data to ask analytic questions towards improving patient outcomes. The final chapter capitalizes on these techniques to not only utilize data to empower improvement in others, but to empower and change yourself.

Empowering yourself begins with the confidence to speak up and know what you're talking about. While speaking up when the topic is "statistics" may be intimidating, the Agency for Healthcare Research and Quality (AHRQ) has found interesting results when asking employees about communication. AHRQ (2016) found that, while speaking up to someone of authority is challenging, speaking up when it impacts patient care is easier. When looking at individual items on the communication openness dimension on the AHRQ safety survey (see Chapter 6 for more information on AHRQ), the nationwide results are high when it comes to speaking up about patient care, but lower when speaking up to others with greater authority. When it comes to questioning the decisions or actions of authority the scores range between 40% and 50%, but when it impacts patient care scores are 70–80% (www.ahrq.gov/sites/default/files/wysiwyg/professionals/quality-patient-safety/patientsafetyculture/hospital/2016/2016_hospitalsops_report_pt2-3.pdf). The only group of respondents who scored above 70% for questioning authority were those in the administrative/ management group. Perhaps this could also explain why non-punitive response to error is within the 40–50% range for all groups except the administrative/ management group. Why can we speak up when it impacts others, but have challenges communicating with authority figures? Is it because you're speaking up for someone else?

A lot of the focus on previous chapters was to teach critical thinking skills to evaluate data and develop interventions to change the behavior of others. What's even more critical is the confidence to speak up by focusing on the FACTS and using the data to empower change in yourself. Data can be a powerful force to not only understand what has happened in the past, but also to determine what can happen in the future. The methodology to analyze the data is as important as the outcome of the story we tell from the data. While data may be used to drive improvement, using techniques to interpret it can change the way you approach data. Together, statistics and research methodology are powerful forces used in storytelling with data. The only limit to what can be achieved is based on your own creativity.

The Art of a Question

When analyzing data and making decisions take a step back and don't jump to conclusions. Changing behavior within others and yourself takes time. Take time to understand the methodology of the process utilized to arrive at the answer. The journey is as much the process as the outcome. Likewise, the knowledge gained through statistics provides more questions than answers. Being able to critically analyze statistics begins with asking the right question. There is an art and skill behind being able to ask the right analytic question and many books exist that provide the skills to ask questions and critically think. Jumping to conclusions without a methodological approach is not the best method for asking questions as it may lead to a focus on gut reactions, hunches, or beliefs based on previous experience; in a way when we are faced with uncomfortable situations we rely on our experience and what we know to move forward. Statistics can invoke fear, which may be the reason why we may ignore the data or facts and make decisions based on experience. Framing the right analytic question is complicated, but an effective approach is three-pronged: creativity, insight, and search.

Think of asking questions as similar to soliciting information from a potential applicant in an interview. The goal of an interview is to obtain as much infor- mation as possible to make the best organizational decision. Analyzing statistics should be treated the same way; it's easy to make assumptions and state beliefs or hunches that appear to be true or confirm a decision you have already made. Remaining objective and focusing on the presented facts promote thinking out- side the box and beyond the meaning of the numbers. The creativity comes from leveraging the formulas used to calculate the statistic, as well as any guidelines/ rules for interpreting patterns/trends. A methodological objective approach to searching for the right question is more effective than subjective hunches.

The first prong is the creative approach to testing your knowledge of statistics. There is no one right way to present data as there are many types of statistics and graphs. Choosing the right statistic to tell the right story to drive change is the difference between storytelling and simply presenting results. It is not challenging to display descriptive statistics and technology makes it easier to create charts/ graphs. However, the real challenge is leveraging the power of statistics to creatively tell a compelling story.

The second prong is utilizing the insight acquired from thinking outside the box and leveraging your knowledge of the statistical formulas to generate additional information. It's relatively easy to become defensive and create excuses, but harder to face the results head on and develop a plan to improve. Many statistical formulas can be used to leverage additional valuable insights. Taking a step back to analyze the components of a formula used to derive a statistic may shed light on some hidden information that may lead to asking a different question.

The third prong is to search for the critical question. Statistics should stimulate more questions than answers. It takes time to search for the right analytic question. It may not be immediately, a day from now, or even a week later, but that light bulb will go off and a question will appear or the original question may generate other questions, causing a need for a deeper dive. Healthcare professionals have a wealth of knowledge and experience resulting in a focus on the right problem, but may be asking the wrong question. Having a plan to STOP and think why the results were presented that way provides a framework to force critical thinking before drawing conclusions.

As technology advances, the amount of metrics and data available increases exponentially, which makes it impossible to know every detail about all metrics. To be able to create change and impact patient care starts with a consistent (reliability) and accurate (validity) process designed to achieve the best possible outcome. Research methodology and statistics are the keys to understanding literature articles or conducting research to advance scientific knowledge. Creating complex solutions may not be sustainable, so keep the process simple. The Three Pillars of Statistics is a conceptual model to categorize the framework for methodological storytelling with data (Figure 10.1).

1. Know your numbers – critically think, evaluate, and DEFINE statistics.
2. Develop behavioral interventions – know how you're being measured and create processes to change behavior through a focus on the FACTS.
3. Set goals to drive change – STOP to develop achievable methodological goals to drive change.

This final chapter methodologically reflects on the concepts learned and develops/enhances skills to critically think and ask the right analytic question to improve employee behavior and patient outcomes and empower yourself. Remember, to change or react to an issue requires a measurement. You can't change what you don't measure, you can't act on what you don't ask, and without data you don't know if change is really happening. Translating numbers into words

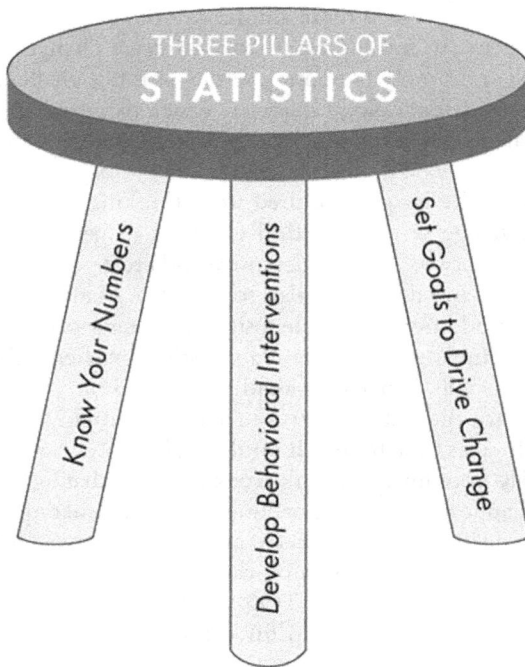

Figure 10.1 Three Pillars of Statistics.

is challenging, but understanding the right questions to ask can lead to the right path for understanding how to improve and promote thinking outside the box.

The Three Pillars of Statistics resulted in the development of the STATISTICS toolkit. This toolkit provides the framework towards a methodological approach to analyzing data or storytelling with data to convey a message effectively. We all have the power to leverage different pictures (Cinderella's castle, Rorschach ink blot, and a control chart) and translate them into stories. These stories may be interpreted differently depending on the individual telling the story and experience/education of the storyteller. Any variation (validity threat) in the story from what is intended is problematic. In the end, there will always be three sides (yours, mine, and reality) to every story, so take the time to methodologically approach data. Remember, the pathway to storytelling with data begins with STATISTICS.

1. Step back and don't jump to conclusions (Chapter 1).
2. Think methodologically (Chapter 2).
3. Analyze the metric (Chapter 3).
4. Test your creativity with understanding the data (Chapter 4).
5. Insights – use the skills learned to question what you see (Chapter 5).
6. Search for the critical questions to ask (Chapter 6).
7. Trending data to understand past, present, and future (Chapter 7).

8. Inquire others to have a complete picture of what is happening (Chapter 8).
9. Conclusions – use all available information to derive conclusions (Chapter 9).
10. Sustainable solutions – create solutions (Chapter 10).

Step 1: Step Back and Don't Jump to Conclusions

Chapter 1 provided an overview of healthcare analytics and the importance of a methodological approach to step back and not jump to conclusions. Often times when faced with problems or desiring to implement change we tend to make decisions based on hunches, beliefs, or previous experience. Change in any industry is inevitable. How an individual responds to change is critical to understanding the best approach to implementing change. There are two extremes individuals may take when viewing change and they are laggards (those resistant to change) and early adopters (those quick to adopting change) (Rogers, 2010). The remainder of individuals fall in the middle. Learning techniques to capitalize on adopting change is the difference between success and failure.

A methodological approach to breaking down a process is an effective means to understand how to improve. When focusing on understanding a process there are always two outcomes: (1) what you think is happening and (2) what is actually happening. We may think that we always know what is going on or the best approach to solve a problem, but this couldn't be further from the truth. Process maps break down the process and highlight the steps followed to understand what is happening. While time may be a factor in emergency healthcare situations, jumping to conclusions without all the facts will not lead to appropriate healthcare interventions. Statistics can be overwhelming, but focusing on improvement/change from a methodological perspective provides structure to focus efforts to change.

Healthcare continues to change and the amount of data to analyze is increasing exponentially. It is very easy to be a victim of information overload. Stepping back and not jumping to conclusions is the moment you need to pause and collect your thoughts before taking action by ensuring you have everything you need to proceed forward. Use a methodological approach to analyzing statistics to break apart an analysis into digestible pieces, so you don't fall victim to jumping to conclusions without the facts.

Step 2: Think Methodologically

Whether consuming information or conducting research, chances are methodology is an integral component to effectively managing change and advancing future knowledge. Within healthcare, plan–do–study–act (PDSA) and root cause analysis (RCA) are two commonly used techniques with similar backgrounds. Both techniques contain step-by-step approaches to ensure implementation is consistent (reliability) and yields accurate (validity) results. Research methodology concepts are disguised with other words, but the prevalence of methodological concepts in healthcare is widely known. The framework of research methodology relies on three different categories of research: experimental design, quasi-experimental design, and non-experimental design. Each research design has its own advantages and disadvantages, but the common framework is a methodological approach to conducting or consuming research. Survey research can be considered a fourth component to research design, but the flexibility of conducting survey research means that it can be any of the three previously mentioned designs. Keep in mind that no one design is better than the other. What's most important is a methodological approach that is consistent (reliable) and accurate (valid).

A methodological approach to a situation leads to a carefully thought-out solution to the problem. There is a methodology to everything. Within statistics, you may not understand the intricacies of every statistics, but using a methodological approach helps to better understand and interpret them. There are two important messages with regards to Chapter 2:

1. How data is measured (nominal, ordinal, interval, and ratio) impacts the type of statistical analysis that can be conducted.
2. DEFINE your metrics.
   D – Denominator – what is your population of interest?
   E – Exclusion criteria – are there any variables that are going to be excluded from your population, sample, or statistic?
   F – Factor – what is it multiplied by? How is your statistic calculated?
   I – Inclusion criteria – are there any variables that are going to be included from your population, sample, or statistic?
   N – Numerator – what part of your population is eligible to be part of the event?
   E – Evaluate all the information to ensure there are no holes in the definition.

The DEFINE tool is an effective methodological approach to begin the process of knowing your numbers. This tool provides a structured approach to interpret any type of statistic or metric to understand how it is being operationalized. Through taking a step back, this tool provides a methodological approach to analyzing statistics.

Step 3: Analyze the Metric

Statistics evoke a variety of different emotions for everyone. Some fear them, others embrace them, and others may be indifferent to them or consider them necessary to make decisions. Regardless of your view, technology has made it possible to analyze large amounts of data to tell a story. When presented with data, it's critically important to analyze the metric and ask questions to ensure a thorough understanding of the calculations used to derive the statistical analysis. There is a difference between knowing your metrics and thinking you know your metrics. Being able to internalize the meaning of the statistics is a step to having the light bulb go off and understanding how to effectively tell the story.

Statistics are complex, but a methodological approach to analyzing statistics breaks down the complexity. Whether the statistics are descriptive or inferential, measures of central tendency or dispersion, parametric or non-parametric, or other higher-level statistical modeling, a systematic approach to analyzing statistics provides the critical information to interpret data or ask questions. A methodological approach to analyzing statistics is accomplished through leveraging the DEFINE tool. This tool ensures a methodological checklist to identify the critical components that comprise any metric (i.e., rate, index, ratio, etc.).

Once the DEFINE tool is used, the next step is to determine the appropriate graphical representation of the statistics to tell the story. Control/run charts are two graphical displays of trended data, and confidence intervals, percentiles/percentile ranks, and odds ratios are statistical concepts that can enhance the story. Statistical significance or a *p* value provides information on whether or not the results are statistically significant. Of equal importance is clinical significance. Keep in mind that metrics can be statistically significant, but not clinically significant or vice versa. Observed rates along with risk-adjusted indices provide two different stories for the same metric. For example, an observed mortality rate tells a story about the actual mortality rate within that particular organization. A risk-adjusted mortality index tells a different story about how the organization is performing compared to others utilizing a regression model. Percentiles and confidence intervals provide further insight into ranking performance to benchmarks or statistical significance. Regardless of what statistics you are analyzing, an understanding of them combined with incorporating different types of statistics results in an effective, compelling, and powerful story.

The following is the DEFINE tool applied to a chronic obstructive pulmonary disease (COPD) readmission rate:

- Denominator – all patients who have COPD.
- Exclusion criteria – expirations, planned readmission, or left against medical advice (AMA). The rationale behind patient exclusions can be based on governmental agencies, literature articles, or clinical expertise.
- Factor – multiply by 100 to convert the value to a percentage.
- Inclusion criteria – expand the denominator to include *International Classification of Diseases* (ICD) diagnosis codes for COPD. Reference AHRQ, the Joint Commission, literature articles, or Centers for Medicare/Medicaid Services (CMS) for how various patient populations are defined.
- Numerator – all patients with index admission of COPD who were readmitted to the hospital within 30 days for any reason.
- Evaluate – this may be a good reminder to think about the scale of measurement. The numerator consists of two outcomes: readmitted or not readmitted. This is converted to a rate, which means the scale of measurement is nominal. Don't confuse the rate with the ratio due to the percentage.

Step 4: Test Your Creativity with Understanding the Data

There is more behind the statistics than the numbers being presented. Every statistic is calculated based on a specific formula. These formulas are useful in understanding how to push the limits of maximizing information to draw conclusions. Take the time to understand the formulas used to derive the statistics and a little creativity to maximize the power behind storytelling with data. At this point, the process of integrating research methodology (Chapter 2) and statistics (Chapter 3) begins with exploring mortality and readmission using graphical representations, such as run charts and control charts.

The importance of focusing on mortality and readmission is a result of hospital performance and financial penalties/incentives that are part of these two metrics and knowing these metrics are part of multiple governmental programs. Implementing change is accomplished through monitoring process and outcome metrics. A process metric is defined as the methods used to arrive at a particular outcome or "how you do something." The outcome metric is defined as the end result of following a process or "how well you did something." These two categories of metrics are intertwined. As hospital performance and financial penalties/incentives are based on outcome metrics, impacting an outcome metric starts with changing a process metric. Driving any type of change begins with understanding the story told utilizing statistics. When analyzing trends, don't forget to focus on the FACTS.

- F: Formulas – identify the formulas for the calculation of the statistics presented.
- A: Analyze patterns/trends – examine variability within the data.
- C: Consider guidelines/rules – determine any guidelines/rules for interpretation.
- T: Think – take time to think about what the data is objectively showing.
- S: Statistics – determine the statistics being used to test your creativity.

Within Chapter 4, the discussion on control charts for trending data focused on the formula for standard deviation. This is where your creativity is tested with the knowledge obtained from the formula for standard deviation, in which the denominator is the sample size. Knowing the influence that sample size has on the standard deviation is important. A smaller sample size results in a larger standard deviation and a larger sample size results in a smaller standard deviation. Knowing this insight can lead to asking different questions.

Think about a control chart and interpreting special cause variation for mortality. It might be tempting to focus on why the mortality rate was above 3 SD for that month (special cause variation). The logical direction would be to review the mortalities (i.e., the outcome) to better understand why there was a high number of deaths in a given month. Knowing the relationship between sample size and standard deviation could transition the focus from the outcome (i.e., mortality) to the process (i.e., more discharges). Can the increase in deaths be attributed to a larger volume of patients for that given month? Or why was there a sudden increase/decrease in patients compared to previous months?

The second example of testing your creativity came from percentile rank in Chapter 5. Focusing on the FACTS and understanding the statistics/formulas provide objective information for interpretation. Recall from Chapter 3 that a percentile rank is used to provide a comparison or benchmark to a larger dataset. This statistic determines how well/poorly an organization is performing. For example, patient satisfaction scores in the 10th percentile indicate performance is better than 10% of other organizations or 90% of organizations are performing better.

To test your creativity further, focus on breaking apart the formula used to calculate the percentile rank. A percentile rank is derived from a score. The score is created from an individual response to a survey. This individual response is rated on a 5-point Likert-type scale where the 1–5 scale is converted to percentages, such that 1 is equal to a score of 0%, 2 is a score of 25%, 3 is a score of 50%, 4 is a score of 75%, and 5 is a score of 100%. If the vendor provides the 50th percentile score, then knowing these FACTS provides additional information. Hypothetically, if the 50th percentile rank equals a score of 89.7, then the average rating is between 4, which is 75, and 5, which is 100. Any individual rating less than 5 contributes to a reduction in the rate. The actual impact on the reduction in the rate is contingent on two factors: (1) how low the rating is on the 5-point Likert-type scale; and (2) sample size included in the analysis. A score of 1 would factor 0% into the calculation of the overall score. Additionally, a smaller sample size would mean that one response would influence the overall score more than a larger sample size.

In the end, it's important to objectively focus on the FACTS and not subjective hunches/beliefs when interpreting any metric or graph. Any statistical analysis should answer some questions, but result in more questions than answers. Understanding statistics is one hurdle, but another is to leverage statistics to drive improvement.

Step 5: Insights – Use the Skills Learned to Question What You See

Results from statistics generate two varied responses: (1) become defensive and create excuses; (2) ask more questions with fewer answers. Regardless of the response, the ambiguity in interpretation is a result of responding to metrics that cannot be directly observed or measured, which are referred to as latent variables. Patient experience is a latent variable, because many factors influence a patient's experience. What can be done is focusing on components of patient experience that can be measured, such as a patient's satisfaction with their nurse/physician, communication, etc. All these factors are operationalized to develop measures that assess the overall construct of patient experience.

The question is: how do we improve a latent variable? A graphical representation of a metric or statistic provides valuable insights in terms of what questions to ask to further analyze the results. Think about any RCA and how many times you ask "why?" to get to the root of the problem. The purpose of presenting statistics is to answer some questions, but having an insight into statistics leads to thought-provoking questions.

Focusing on the FACTS with standard deviation in the control chart revealed the denominator of formula is the sample size. As a result, a large standard deviation may indicate a change in volume or sample size. Before jumping to conclusions and asking why there was a change in volume, take a minute to reflect on your own insight. Suggesting a change in volume can impact financial reimbursement may lead others down the wrong path for improvement. Instead of jumping to conclusions, what other explanations (i.e., internal validity) could cause a decrease in volume? Could a decrease in volume for a particular metric be a result of shifting services to another organization or no longer offering that type of service? Perhaps there are some high-volume inpatient surgeries being done as an outpatient, which may impact volume.

Subjective information could generate significant criticisms that deflect from the story and result in creating excuses or becoming defensive. Providing the FACTS of the analysis is more challenging to debate and question. The only way to move from hunches/beliefs of a phenomenon of interest is through the incorporation of objective facts. A methodological approach would be to reflect on the statistics presented and experience within the organization to generate insightful ideas that are the basis for analytic questions.

Step 6: Search for the Critical Questions to Ask

Be realistic and know that it's not possible to have all the answers to every problem. It takes time to search for the right analytic question to ask. Relying on a methodological approach ensures all statistics are approached in the same manner. STOP and develop a plan to achieve the desired goal. For example, Chapter 6 contains the AHRQ safety survey. There are many constructs defined in the survey with many paths towards improvement. Implementing everything is not effective, so take the time to plan and think.

In reviewing all the domains, consider the handoffs and transitions domain. When analyzing the domain, the purpose of any statistical analysis is to know how the construct is defined. Jumping to conclusions and taking action without understanding the definition can lead to the wrong question being asked. A methodological approach to defining metrics reveals that AHRQ defines handoffs and transitions based on two questions assessing shift changes and two questions assessing transfer of information. Think of it this way: if employees rate all 5s for the shift change questions and all 1s for the transfer of information, then the overall average is 3. The meaning of the domain is hidden in the details.

A further focus group is needed to better understand what specific aspects of handoffs and transitions employees were thinking of when responding to those questions. Nothing can be fixed if the implemented intervention doesn't address the questions being measured. Are the questions related to shift changes or transfer of information within the same department or across departments? Not knowing the answer to this critical question will result in an intervention that may not improve the domain. The STOP tool provides a framework to focus on the critical question to ask through understanding the plan of what to accomplish.

- S – SMART goal – determining what question to ask begins with understanding the goal of where to improve.
- T – Think critically – leverage the skills learned about analyzing metrics and test your creativity with understanding the presented data.

- O – Operationalization of your metrics – thinking from a methodological perspective about how variables are defined (i.e., construct validity) helps to better understand how a metric is being measured.
- P – Purpose – when determining what questions to ask, the purpose could be to develop behavioral interventions or set a goal to impact a future performance penalty/incentive.

Changing any type of behavior doesn't come without challenges. Thinking through the process and understanding how others react/resist change are key to developing an intervention with lasting improvement. To illustrate how this tool works, a patient experience question related to likelihood to recommend will be used.

- SMART goal – achieve the 90th percentile for likelihood to recommend in 5 years.
- Think critically – percentile ranks, observed scores, and individual ratings on a Likert-type scale are all important to understand how to improve. Need to understand the complexity of how likelihood to recommend is defined and measured.
- Operationalization of your metrics – taking a moment to DEFINE likelihood to recommend will provide insight into how this metric is being measured.
- Purpose – conduct a focus group with patients to understand the interpretation of likelihood to recommend (i.e., what do they think about?). Determine how to trend data over time. Isolate the key components to improving likelihood to recommend ensuring no other explanation or intervention occurs that could explain any changes. To impact the future CMS Star Rating.

Scoring the likelihood to recommend question is complex. The end result is a comparative percentile rank to others within the database, but the story of how the percentile rank is created is critical. The percentile rank is comprised of a score ranging between 0 and 100. To calculate these scores, a 1–5-point Likert-type scale is anchored with five responses that are converted to 0, 25, 50, 75, and 100 points, and an overall average is calculated.

Consider the following example using fictitious numbers. The 25th percentile for likelihood to recommend corresponds to score of 87.2. Assume the 50th percentile rank converts to a score of 87.6. A patient rating of 4 equals a score of 75 and a rating of 5 equals a score of 100. With an average score of 87.2, any survey response below 5 results in a decrease in the overall average and percentile rank. Additionally, take into consideration the monthly sample size and how much of an influence one response could have on the overall average. The SMART goal was to achieve the 90th percentile within 5 years with the emphasis on focus groups to understand how patients interpret this item and then isolate the key components to build into an intervention. To move from the SMART goal to a plan requires research methodology and statistics to generate the question. A starting question could be: what will it take for a patient to rate a 5 instead of a 4? A carefully crafted question provides the critical information to understand what is happening now and how to change the future.

Step 7: Trending Data to Understand Past, Present, and Future

The best predictor of future performance is past behavior (Wernimont & Campbell, 1968), so there's no question of the value of trending the past and present to understand where the future may go. This step is a transition from analyzing individual statistics towards trending data to graphically enhance the story. Data is a powerful tool to understand what happened in the past, what is currently happening, and what could happen in the future. With the enhancement of technology, monitoring trends in real time allows for taking action faster, but don't forget to step back and not jump to conclusions too quickly. Through trended data, complex analyses (i.e., predictive analytics) can be used to understand how to impact the future. Part of the future is unknown and is subject to change at a rapid pace depending on governmental initiatives, the direction CMS may take with various initiatives related to performance and financial incentives/penalties, and healthcare organization priorities. Being proactive instead of reactive is a way to stay ahead of moving targets.

Regardless of what the future holds, trending data over time is a means to monitor trends and patterns within metrics. A few different approaches to presenting data have been presented from run charts and control charts (Chapter 4 – mortality and readmission), bar charts with percentile ranks graphed (Chapter 5 – patient experience), bar charts and crosstabs (Chapter 6 – AHRQ safety survey), statistics to project into the future (Chapter 7 – past, present, and future), interactive dashboards (Chapter 8 – CMS Star Rating), and dashboards with confidence intervals plotted (Chapter 9 – CMS Hospital Compare). The only right way to present data is one that generates stories to drive change and stimulate discussions.

Step 8: Inquire Others to Have a Complete Picture of What is Happening

Publicly reported data and increased competition bring up interesting and new questions. Staying focused on internal improvements is important, but what is happening outside the four walls of the organization is critical to improving performance and hit those moving targets. Being internal to an organization means focusing on processes and outcomes within control. This is no longer a sustainable solution as the present and future focus on improving patient outcomes driven by financial and performance metrics defined by outside performance. Staying focused on internal efforts without considering external expertise has the potential to result in groupthink. Groupthink is a psychological concept where groups comprised of similar backgrounds make erroneous decisions based on no one individual being willing to speak up out of a desire to conform to the group (Janis, 1972). Organizations may not have all the answers to solve every problem, so take a step back and see what best practices are happening outside your four walls.

Relying on patterns/trends will only suffice for a short period of time. Recognize that no one person has all the answers, so whether it's analyzing data for patterns/trends, defining metrics, focusing on the facts of the data presented, or examining government or state initiatives to stay ahead of the changes, there is only so much that one person can be responsible for. Think outside the box and inquire with others outside your department, hospital, or organization; they may provide answers or drive further questions to hit those moving targets. Drawing conclusions takes time and one mistake could result in a loss of time, money, and motivation. A systematic approach would be to develop solutions by not jumping to conclusions and focusing on asking the right questions. An example of why it's important to inquire what others are doing is the data that CMS provides for the star rating. The CMS Star Rating is a performance comparison of all hospitals across a variety of metrics and is available publicly. The moral of the story is that healthcare is increasingly competitive. Patients are more analytically savvy and making more informed decisions on where they *choose* to receive care.

The question is, "will you take the step to leverage the power that statistics have to tell a story with data and hit those moving targets?" Most stories should drive more questions than answers. One technique to dive deeper, assuming time and resources are available, is to conduct focus groups. Focus groups are an excellent way of being able to inquire of others as to what is currently happening and provide an alternative perspective of where to go next or create a process map to drive change.

Conducting focus groups provides insightful information about how others perceive information and reflect on questions being asked. The following discussion is a focus group that took place in two different hospitals containing 10–30 healthcare professions. The topic of the focus group was patient experience and how to improve likelihood to recommend. The conversation began with a simple question of, "what do patients mean when they respond to the question how likely would you recommend this hospital?" What were they thinking about? Was it the nurse/physician communication? Cleanliness of their room? Any issues in the emergency department? Or temperature of their food? The truth is that any of these questions could influence a patient's likelihood to recommend. It is possible that from a survey methodology perspective patients were primed to respond to the likelihood to recommend question on the basis of the questions that are around this question. After this short discussion came to an end, the entire group collectively said, "we should ask the patients." This short example illustrates the importance of asking the right question and empowering others through inquiring what they know. The answer to the question may not come from your colleagues or administration, but rather from the person to whom the service is directly provided.

The moral of the story is that there are many available tools to ensure organizational success. The key is capitalizing on these tools to drive sustainable and consistent improvement. The pathway to hitting moving targets is not accomplished alone. Leverage the knowledge and skills by inquiring what others are doing and the present/future direction of governmental and state initiatives that may have financial or performance incentives/penalties.

Step 9: Conclusions – Use All Available Information to Derive Conclusions

Taking a shortcut or heuristic to rely on hunches or beliefs may not result in driving sustainable improvement. Using heuristics based on experience may make processes easier, but because something is easier doesn't mean it is the right approach. The process of analyzing statistics is as critical as the outcome of those results. A multi-faceted approach to analyzing data includes a methodological approach to statistics to effectively tell a story with data that drives change. Once all statistical data has been collected and analyzed along with using any necessary tools (i.e., DEFINE, FACTS, STOP, etc.) to generate quantitative and qualitative data, the process of storytelling with data and deriving conclusions begins.

The overall conclusions drawn from any type of statistics lead to alternative explanations (i.e., threats to validity). Having the tools and skill set to question the displayed results leads to a greater internalization of the presented metrics. Creating excuses, becoming defensive, or deflecting the story told by statistics doesn't solve the problem. Taking time to understand and appreciate statistics and research methodology improves decision making and generates an understanding of the presented results. The pathway to storytelling with data begins with statistics and ends with a proactive approach to hitting those moving targets. This interpretation involves the ability and skill to recognize the type of statistics presented, understand what it means, and effectively interpret them to develop the insight to ask the right question to assess, monitor, and drive improvement efforts.

Prior to moving towards developing sustainable interventions or solutions, it's important to reflect on what has been discussed. Matejka and Fitzmaurice (2017) developed 12 different visual displays of data with identical statistical properties, highlighting that multiple graphical representations result in different stories, which leads to questions of doubt and opens up opportunities for criticism. Statistics provide quantitative facts. It's what is done with them that creates confusion/uncertainty. Statistics in the wrong hands or used incorrectly lead to skepticism, generating excuses and/or blame or focusing on the wrong solution. Used appropriately, statistics are powerful tools that provide value to monitoring and driving improvement.

Step 10: Sustainable Solutions – Create Solutions

The process to analyzing statistics isn't hard. The hard part is consistently and accurately following the steps to methodologically approach every analysis and avoiding heuristics to complete a task quicker. While drawing conclusions from results is complicated, developing sustainable solutions is even more challenging. Implementing change or improvement that is sustainable and that will be followed by everyone all the time is the key to hitting those moving targets. Empower yourself to draw conclusions and develop appropriate solutions to drive sustainable change through incorporating behavioral interventions, all while focusing on the facts of the data.

There is no "one size fits all" approach for developing sustainable solutions. The psychological aspect of human behavior suggests that changes in behavior result from personality, motivation, leadership, cognitive theories, behavioral theories, etc. When a process is misaligned to behavior, the chances of a successful process diminish, and the former process/behavior emerges. Within the realm of psychology and human behavior when making decisions it's common to develop heuristics. Whenever a process is developed there will likely be others looking for these mental shortcuts to accomplish work either more efficiently or quicker, or leave out unnecessary steps. While the STATISTICS toolkit is a 10-step process to interpreting analytics, all steps within the process naturally build on each other. The three developed tools incorporate aspects of each of the STATISTICS toolkit and the Three Pillars of Statistics conceptual framework provides the backbone to guide and interpret analytics.

Everyone is motivated to achieve success in a different way. Every decision or intervention developed is similar to a fork in the road. Some may go down one path, some may go down others, and some may forge their own path. Handling change and steering an organization towards moving targets are enormous responsibilities. There will be points of discouragement and disappointment, but chances of success can't happen without failure. Failure and mistakes are just reminders that you haven't found the right path to success. The purpose of this book was to provide insight into an alternative approach built on integrating research methodology and statistics with healthcare data, resulting in effective storytelling. Creating solutions with a methodological focus on process and outcome, understanding how to effectively tell a story with data, and making mistakes are all part of learning. We don't have all the answers, but together we can impact change.

In closing, the journey of storytelling with STATISTICS is just the beginning. The Three Pillars of Statistics conceptual framework provides the foundation to know your numbers, develop behavioral interventions, and set goals to drive change. These aims, when combined, are pillars that lay the foundation to analyzing statistics to tell a story. Take the time to *step* back and don't jump to conclusions through *thinking* methodologically. DEFINE and *analyze* metrics to *test* your creative *insight* while focusing on the FACTS. *Searching* for the right analytic question to effectively *trend* data takes time, so don't forget to STOP and think outside the box. *Inquire* with others to gain a different perspective prior to drawing *conclusions* and remember to develop *sustainable* solutions. While our journey is coming to an end, we hope this inspires you to look at data in a different way and helps you with your journey to storytelling with STATISTICS.

Discussion Questions

- Think of a time when you had to communicate a difficult message. What did you do that went well? What were your opportunities to improve?
- Think about the last time you asked a question by jumping to conclusions. With hindsight being 20/20, what do you know now that could have caused you to ask the question differently?

- As a result of this book, name one thing that you will do differently when analyzing data.
- What benefits do you see in using the DEFINE, FACTS, and STOP tools to guide improvement?

Glossary

alpha, alpha level, *p* value, or α   the likelihood or probability that the results of the experiment are due to chance

Applied research   research that aims to answer questions from real-world or organizational problems

Astronomical point   an unusually large or small point of data

Bar graph   a graph using rectangular bars that display the value of a certain metric

Basic research   research that aims to find answers to questions we do not have the answers to

Beta or β   the probability or percent chance of making a type II error

Bipolar scale   a measurement scale representing both sides of measurement of interest. For example, extremely dissatisfied to extremely satisfied

Cluster sampling   dividing the population into groups or clusters by geographical location, for example, and then selecting a random sample

Confidence intervals   a range of values that a certain parameter may fall within

Confounding variable   a variable that was unaccounted for in a study that may alter the results of the study

Construct validity   the measures intended to be represented actually measure what they are intended to measure

Continuous variables   variables that are either interval or ratio

Control chart   a graph that displays data over time, including the upper and lower control limits (typically displayed as standard deviations)

Convenience sampling   selecting the sample based on who you have access to

Correlational design   a research design that seeks to find relationships among variables

Criterion variable   the outcome variable being predicted in regression

Descriptive statistics   designed to describe or summarize data

Dichotomous variable   a variable with two outcomes, generally a 1 or 0

Evidence-based practice   utilizes a problem-solving approach to incorporate the best evidence in the literature, patient preferences, and clinical expertise to make decisions

Extraneous variable a variable that is not intended to be measured in a study

Factor loading a measure of the variance of a variable on a specific factor

Generalizability the extension of findings from data taken from a sample population to the entire population

Geometric mean also known as the median, can be used in place of the arithmetic mean

Inadequate explication of constructs the definition is vague or not completely clear, where individuals interpret the definition in different ways

Index created when the denominator is large, so the calculation is a numerator divided by a denominator multiplied by 1,000

Inferential statistics designed to infer or deduce information from data

Internal consistency, coefficient alpha, or Cronbach's apla reliability a measure of how similar items on a test measure the same construct

Interquartile range the final measure of dispersion where a dataset is divided into quartiles split by the 25th, 50th, and 75th percentiles

Interrater reliability different raters or people rating the same metric

Intrarater reliability same rater or person rating the same metric over time

k-means clustering mathematically assigns a ranking, or in this case, a star rating, to combine multiple metrics assessed on different scales of measurement

Latent variable a variable that cannot be directly observed or measured

Linear regression predicts a continuous outcome or a variable on an interval or ratio scale

Logistic regression predicts categorical/dichotomous outcomes or nominal scales of measurement

Manifest variable a variable tha can be directly observed or measured

Mean the average and most widely reported measure of central tendency

Median the number in the middle of a dataset

Measure loading a measure of the variance of a variable on a specific measure

Metrics a variable that is measured and tracked

Mode the number that appears the most often in a dataset

Non-experimental research research that does not use manipulations and/ or does not use random sampling

Non-parametric statistics does not have the restriction of relying on normally distributed data

Non-probability sampling a range of sampling techniques that do not randomly select participants

Non-response bias occurs when there may be differences between participants who respond to a survey compared to those who did not

Odds ratio interpreted as a measure of probability or a measure of association between two things

Operationalization the process of defining something

Outcome metrics outcome metrics focus on the end result of what happened when something was done

Outliers values that are well above or below the average

Parametric statistics   relies on normally distributed data

Pareto chart   a graph, similar to a bar graph, but that shows values in descending order like that of a Pareto distribution

Percentile ranks/percentiles   the amount of scores (typically described as percentiles) in a frequency distribution that are equal to or lower than that score

Pie chart   a graph where a circle is divided into prortions representing different metrics

Power   the chance of finding statistical significance

Probability sampling   a range of sampling techniques that randomly selects participants

Process metrics   focusing on the steps conducted to accomplish something

Purposive sampling   selecting a sample based on a specific criterion that is relevant to the research question of interest (i.e., selecting females for a study on women's health)

p **value**   the likelihood or probability that the results of the experiment are due to chance

Qualitative scales of measurement   measures that use nominal and ordinal data

Quantitative scales of measurement   measures that use interval and ratio data

Quasi-experimental research   research that aims to find cause-and-effect relationships among variables without using random sampling

Quota sampling   similar to stratified sampling, where a population is divided into subgroups. The difference is being told how many individuals to collect data from based on a criterion of interest

Random assignment   a sampling method where each potential participant has an equal opportunity to be selected

Range   a crude measure of variability calculated by subtracting the largest and smallest value in a dataset

Rate   a numerator divided by a denominator multiplied by 100

Rating errors   intended or unintended biases when completing survey items

Ratio   a comparison between two non-zero values

Regression   a statistical technique that desires to predict an outcome

Reliability   the extent to which a measure in a study is consistent, dependable, precise, or stable

Reliability coefficient   the unit of measurement that describes the reliability of a measure

Response rate   the total number of participants who took the survey/ questionnaire divided by the overall sample

Reverse-scored item   rephrasing a statement or question so that the scale used to measure that statement or question is reversed

Risk-adjusted measure   an observed rate divided by an expected rate where the expected rate is adjusted using a complex logistic regression model (see Chapter 3 for further information)

Run   a series of data points above or below the mean line

Run chart   a graph that displays data over time

Sampling   the process of collecting participants for research projects

Scatter plot   a graph where the values of two variables are plotted along two intersecting axes

Shift   a series of six or more consecutive points that are all either above or below the mean line

Simple random sampling   using a random number generator, such as the Rand() function in Microsoft Excel, to randomly select your sample

Skewed   not normally distributed

Snowball sampling   selecting a sample where current participants are used to obtain additional participants (i.e., using a participant with a rare condition to find others with the same condition)

Standard deviation   a measure of variability or spread of a data set around the mean that is measured in the same units as the calculated measure. It is calculated by the square root of the variance

Stratified sampling   dividing the population into subgroups, or strata (i.e., nurses and physicians, or administrative, clinical, and non-clinical), and selecting a random sample

Translational research   a process with a multidisciplinary approach to integrate research conducted in the lab to develop new ways to treat in practice

Trend   a series of five or more points that are all increasing or decreasing

Type I error   stating that there is significance when there isn't

Type II error   stating no significant difference is found, but there actually is significance

Unipolar scale   a measurement scale representing one side of measurement of interest and 0 point for the other. For example, not at all satisfied to completely satisfied

Validity   the accuracy of a measure

Validity coefficient   the unit of measurement that describes the accuracy of a measure

Variance   difference between an observed value and an expected value or a measure of variability around a mean.

z-score distribution   a distribution where scores indicate the amount of standard deviations the score is above or below the mean

References

AHRQ. (2016). *Hospital Survey on Patient Safety Culture.* Retrieved from: www.ahrq.gov/ sites/default/files/wysiwyg/professionals/quality-patient-safety/patientsafetyculture/ hospital/2016/2016_hospitalsops_report_pt1.pdf

Armstrong, J. S., & Overton, T. S. (1977). Estimating nonresponse bias in mail surveys. *Journal of Marketing Research, 14(3),* 396–402.

Azoulay, É., Pochard, F., Chevret, S., Adrie, C., Annane, D., Bleichner, G., ... & Goldgran-Toledano, D. (2004). Half the family members of intensive care unit patients do not want to share in the decision-making process: A study in 78 French intensive care units. *Critical Care Medicine, 32*(9), 1832–1838.

Bandura, A. (1991). Social cognitive theory of self-regulation. *Organizational Behavior and Human Decision Processes, 50*(2), 248–287.

Barclay, S., Todd, C., Finlay, I., Grande, G., & Wyatt, P. (2002). Not another questionnaire! Maximizing the response rate, predicting non-response and assessing non-response bias in postal questionnaire studies of GPs. *Family Practice, 19(1),* 105–111.

Barnette, J. J. (2000). Effects of stem and Likert response option reversals on survey internal consistency: If you feel the need, there is a better alternative to using those negatively worded stems. *Educational and Psychological Measurement, 60*(3), 361–370.

Barry, M. J., & Edgman-Levitan, S. (2012). Shared decision making – The pinnacle patient-centered care. *New England Journal of Medicine, 366*(9), 780–781.

Bergomi, G. (2014). The Joint Commission and Cleveland Clinic reducing colorectal surgical site infections. Presentation at NSQIP Conference.

Berwick, D. M. (2009). What 'patient-centered' should mean: Confessions of an extremist: A seasoned clinician and expert fears the loss of his humanity if he should become a patient. *Health Affairs, 28*(Suppl. 1), w555–w565.

Blegen, M. A., Gearhart, S., O'Brien, R., Sehgal, N. L., & Alldredge, B. K. (2009). AHRQ's hospital survey on patient safety culture: Psychometric analyses. *Journal of Patient Safety, 5*(3), 139–144.

Bleich, S. N., Özaltin, E., & Murray, C. J. (2009). How does satisfaction with the health-care system relate to patient experience? *Bulletin of the World Health Organization, 87*(4), 271–278.

Brutus, S., Gill, H., & Duniewicz, K. (2010). State of science in industrial and organizational psychology: A review of self-reported limitations. *Personnel Psychology, 63*, 907–936.

Classen, D. C., Pestotnik, S. L., Evans, R. S., Lloyd, J. F., & Burke, J. P. (1997). Adverse drug events in hospitalized patients: Excess length of stay, extra costs, and attributable mortality. *JAMA, 277*(4), 301–306.

Cohen, J. (1988). *Statistical power analysis for the behavioral sciences* (2nd ed.). Mahwah, NJ: Erlbaum.

Cook, C., Heath, F., & Thompson, R. L. (2000). A meta-analysis of response rates in web- or internet-based surveys. *Educational and Psychological Measurement, 60(6)*, 821–836.

Cronbach, L. J. (1951). Coefficient alpha and the internal structure of tests. *Psychometrika, 16(3)*, 297–334.

DiCuccio, M. H. (2015). The relationship between patient safety culture and patient outcomes: A systematic review. *Journal of Patient Safety, 11(3)*, 135–142.

Dillman, D. A. (2007). *Mail and internet surveys: The tailored design method* (2nd ed.). Hoboken, NJ: Wiley.

Epstein, R. M., & Street, R. L. (2011). The values and value of patient-centered care. Annals of Family Medicine, *9(2)*, 100–103.

Field, A. (2017). *Discovering Statistics Using SPSS: North American Edition.* 5th edition. Thousand Oaks, CA: Sage Publications.

Frampton, S., Guastello, S., Brady, C., Hale, M., Horowitz, S., Bennett Smith, S., & Stone, S. (2008). *Patient-centered care improvement guide.* Derby, CT: Planetree.

Fulton, B. R. (2018). Organizations and survey research: Implementing response enhancing strategies and conducting nonresponse analyses. *Sociological Methods & Research, 47(2)*, 240–276.

Godolphin, W. (2009). Shared decision-making. *Healthcare Quarterly, 12*(Sp).

Horan, P. M., DiStefano, C., & Motl, R. W. (2003). Wording effects in self-esteem scales: Methodological artifact or response style? *Structural Equation Modeling, 10(3)*, 435–455.

Huff, D. (1993). *How to lie with statistics.* New York, NY: WW Norton.

Hyman, H. (1944). Do they tell the truth? *The Public Opinion Quarterly, 8(4)*, 557–559.

Janis, I. L. (1972). *Victims of groupthink: A psychological study of foreign-policy decisions and fiascoes.* Boston, MA: Houghton-Mifflin.

Junewicz, A., & Youngner, S. J. (2015). Patient-satisfaction surveys on a scale of 0 to 10: Improving health care, or leading it astray? *Hastings Center Report, 45(3)*, 43–51.

Kaplowitz, M. D., Hadlock, T. D., & Levine, R. (2004). A comparison of web and mail survey response rates. *Public Opinion Quarterly, 68(1)*, 94–101.

Kivits, J. (2006). Informed patients and the internet: A mediated context for consultations with health professionals. *Journal of Health Psychology, 11(2)*, 269–282.

Likert, R. A. (1932). A technique for the measurement of attitudes. *Archives of Psychology, 140,* 1–55.

Locke, E. A., & Latham, G. P. (1990). *A theory of goal setting and task performance.* Englewood Cliffs, NJ: Prentice-Hall.

Lutsky, L. A., Risucci, D. A., & Tortolani, A. J. (1993). Reliability and accuracy of surgical resident peer ratings. *Evaluation Review, 17(4)*, 444–456.

Manary, M. P., Boulding, W., Staelin, R., & Glickman, S. W. (2013). The patient experience and health outcomes. *New England Journal of Medicine, 368(3)*, 201–203.

Mardon, R. E., Khanna, K., Sorra, J., Dyer, N., & Famolaro, T. (2010). Exploring relationships between hospital patient safety culture and adverse events. *Journal of Patient Safety, 6(4)*, 226–232.

Matejka, J., & Fitzmaurice, G. (2017, May). Same stats, different graphs: Generating datasets with varied appearance and identical statistics through simulated annealing. In *Proceedings of the 2017 CHI Conference on Human Factors in Computing Systems* (pp. 1290–1294).

Mazaheri, M., & Theuns, P. (2009). Effects of varying response formats on self-ratings of life-satisfaction. *Social Indicators Research, 90(3)*, 381.

Miller, G. A. (1956). The magical number seven, plus or minus two: Some limits on our capacity for processing information. *Psychological Review. 63 (2)*: 81–97.

More Than a Gut Feeling. (video). Retrieved from: www.media-partners.com/interviewing_training_videos/more_than_a_gut_feeling_iv.htm?h1=&utm_source=google&utm_medium=cpc&utm_campaign=all-mp-produced-films&utm_content=mtagf-more-than-a-gut-feeling&utm_term=more%20than%20a%20gut%20feeling&gclid=CjwKCAjwzIH7BRAbEiwAoDxxTkYMUfS3DQoZJdcC-dgVJhewlVjdCeSahZYDxu7ldEUjzjeUVpoFUxoC010QAvD_BwE

Muchinsky, P. M. (2006). *Psychology applied to work: An introduction to industrial and organizational psychology.* Belmont, CA: Cengage Learning.

Naylor, A. R., & Ricco, J. B. (2013). The story of anybody, somebody, nobody and everybody. *European Journal of Vascular and Endovascular Surgery, 46*(5), 506–507.

Nimon, K., Shuck, B., & Zigarmi, D. (2016). Construct overlap between employee engagement and job satisfaction: A function of semantic equivalence? *Journal of Happiness Studies, 17*(3), 1149–1171.

Ong, A. D., & Weiss, D. J. (2000). The impact of anonymity on responses to sensitive questions 1. *Journal of Applied Social Psychology, 30*(8), 1691–1708.

Ouellette, J. A., & Wood, W. (1998). Habit and intention in everyday life: The multiple processes by which past behavior predicts future behavior. *Psychological Bulletin, 124(1),* 54.

Parikh, S., George, P., Liyanage-Don, N., Hohler, A., Denis, R., & Weinberg, J. (2017). Hospital readmissions following stroke: A retrospective study (P6.270). Presented in poster format at the American Academy of Neurology Annual Meeting in Boston, MA.

Picardi, C. A., & Masick, K. D. (2013). *Research methods: Designing and conducting research with a real-world focus.* Thousand Oaks, CA: Sage.

Provost, L. P., & Murray, S. (2011). *The Health Care Data Guide: Learning from data for improvement.* San Francisco, CA: Jossey Bass.

Reynolds, A. (2009). Patient-centered care. *Radiologic Technology, 81*(2), 133–147.

Rogers, E. M. (2010). *Diffusion of innovations.* New York, NY: Simon and Schuster.

Rubin, H. R., Pronovost, P., & Diette, G. B. (2001). The advantages and disadvantages of process-based measures of health care quality. *International Journal for Quality in Health Care, 13*(6), 469–474.

Russell, J. A., & Carroll, J. M. (1999). On the bipolarity of positive and negative affect. *Psychological Bulletin, 125*(1), 3.

Shadish, W. R., Cook, T. D., & Campbell, D. T. (2002). *Experimental and quasi-experimental designs for generalized causal inference.* Boston, MA: Houghton Mifflin.

Small, D., & Small, R. (2011). Patients first! Engaging the hearts and minds of nurses with a patient-centered practice model. *OJIN: The Online Journal of Issues in Nursing, 16*(2), 109–120.

Sorra, J. S., & Dyer, N. (2010). Multilevel psychometric properties of the AHRQ hospital msurvey on patient safety culture. *BMC Health Services Research, 10*(1), 199.

Trzeciak, S., Gaughan, J. P., Bosire, J., & Mazzarelli, A. J. (2016). Association between Medicare summary star ratings for patient experience and clinical outcomes in US hospitals. *Journal of Patient Experience, 3*(1), 6–9.

Vautier, S., & Pohl, S. (2009). Do balances scales assess bipolar constructs? *Psychological Assessment, 21*(2), 187–193.

Vautier, S., Callahan, S., Moncany, D., & Sztulman, H. (2004). A bistable view of single constructs measured using balanced questionnaires: Application to trait anxiety. *Structural Equation Modeling, 11*(2), 261–271.

Vogus, T. J., Sutcliffe, K. M., & Weick, K. E. (2010). Doing no harm: Enabling, enacting, and elaborating a culture of safety in health care. *Academy of Management Perspectives, 24*(4), 60–77.

Waterworth, S., & Luker, K. A. (1990). Reluctant collaborators: Do patients want to be involved in decisions concerning care? *Journal of Advanced Nursing, 15*(8), 971–976.

Weaver, S. J., Lubomksi, L. H., Wilson, R. F., Pfoh, E. R., Martinez, K. A., & Dy, S. M. (2013). Promoting a culture of safety as a patient safety strategy: A systematic review. *Annals of Internal Medicine, 158*(5), 369–374.

Wernimont, P. F., & Campbell, J. P. (1968). Signs, samples, and criteria. *Journal of Applied Psychology, 52*(5), 372.

Wildman, R. C. (1977). Effects of anonymity and social setting on survey responses. *Public Opinion Quarterly, 41*(1), 74–79.

Index

Note: Page numbers in *italics* indicate figures and in **bold** indicate tables on the corresponding pages.

For Product Safety Concerns and Information please contact our EU
representative GPSR@taylorandfrancis.com
Taylor & Francis Verlag GmbH, Kaufingerstraße 24, 80331 München, Germany

www.ingramcontent.com/pod-product-compliance
Lightning Source LLC
Chambersburg PA
CBHW070719220326
41598CB00024BA/3236